CLINGING TO HIS WORD
THROUGH CANCER

"Blessed be the God and Father of our Lord Jesus Christ,

the Father of mercies and God of all comfort,

who comforts us in all our affliction,

so that we may be able to comfort those who are in any affliction,

with the comfort with which we ourselves are comforted by God.

For as we share abundantly in Christ's sufferings,

so through Christ we share abundantly in comfort too"

2 Corinthians 1:3-5 (English Standard Version)

LAURA PENTSA

CLINGING TO HIS WORD THROUGH CANCER

Lessons From A Breast Cancer Survivor's Account, Shared For Times Of Trial.

Encouragement and practical advice for the body, mind, and spirit!

LAURA PENTSA

ISBN-10: 1548424684
ISBN-13: 978-1548424688

To my loving family,

Dave, Joel, Leah, and Gabrielle

who have added so much happiness and excitement to my life

LAURA PENTSA

CONTENTS

.

:ACKNOWLEDGMENTS:

I have been incredibly blessed by the support, comfort, friendship and guidance that true loved ones can lend during times of extreme trial and transitions. I was supported in every possible way during my personal battle with triple-negative breast cancer, into survivorship and while writing this book.

Though it would be utterly impossible to thank every person individually by name, I will try to acknowledge the efforts and support poured out on our family by so many!

To my talented friends and family who helped edit and polish this book, I thank you! You've helped me take my lessons and create something beautiful. Dave, you were the one taking care of the kids when I was glued to the computer, typing on and on! You never complained about cereal for dinner when I was inspired to get a thought down. You were the first one I could be vulnerable enough to show these pages, and ask for help. I was scared and nervous to reveal all of my thoughts and put you in a tough spot, but you carefully read it all, and helped me to be better. To my dear friend Deb, you encouraged me through the writing process and helped me believe this was valuable. Your love of books and reading provided a unique talent. You used that gift and gave me a fresh perspective and different point of view, both critical and priceless! To my brother-in-law Mike, thank you for graciously reading through my draft with your keen eye for grammar and detail. To my life long friend Mark, thank you for using your expertise to take my photo and create a beautiful book cover!

From the moment I was diagnosed with cancer I needed support. I must thank Facebook for supplying a mode of communication, that allowed others to know what was happening during my cancer treatment and in return allowed them the opportunity to shower me with encouragement, positivity, and well wishes! The comments that continually came into my Facebook newsfeed were uplifting and brightened my days. Even on lonely sick days in bed, I was able to be surrounded with words of affirmation and support from my many "Facebook Friends".

To the numerous outstanding people I met through Honor Health and various Valley medical practices, I respect and appreciate all of you. The medical treatment I received was top notch! I thank my doctors, nurses, oncology navigator, advisors and all of their medical teams for taking wonderful care of me, providing the medicine my body desperately needed, the surgeries that removed both danger and risks, as well as the stitches and oxygen therapies that brought me healing. Without any one of you, my treatment would not have been complete. Thank you for guiding me through that difficult time with wisdom, knowledge, and compassion!

I'd like to thank the many artists and composers who have dedicated their life's work to creating inspiring, uplifting, Godly music that brings perspective, praise, and worship! I have never been as impacted by song as I was during my cancer journey, and I know Christian music was a critical piece of my healing. Special thanks to Rend Collective and I am They. I worshiped the Lord through your music and experienced great joy through the beautiful lyrics.

I cannot begin to thank all of my church family and friends for their unending love and support for our family! They welcomed us with open arms when we moved to Arizona five years ago, and have been ready and willing to support us in every imaginable way ever since! Providing meals, groceries, babysitting, errands, providing financial support, sitting with us, praying with us and for us! Our fellowship, our home away from home, being our extended family, and our best friends. You have blessed us more than you'll ever know!

Overwhelming thanks to all of our Ohio family who were so eager to help. Sending cards of encouragements, boxes of gifts to me and the family! Sending checks to help with tests and medicine which insurance had declined. For the many who even flew out here to spend time taking care of the kids, helping with the house and being at my side when things got tough! I will never forget the efforts and sacrifices you made showing us love! You made a huge difference in this experience and I am forever grateful!

Special thanks to Mom, Dad and my brother Steve, who would stop by often and check on me, I am thankful that we all lived so close together. Thank you for cheering me on and helping me through some of the most challenging of days. Mom, I cannot imagine what we would have done without you! You sacrificed so much of your time and energy putting our needs ahead of your own. Serving our family with love, even through your own pain, sadness, and exhaustion. Thank you!

Heartfelt thanks to my children, who never treated me any differently. To them I was never a sick patient, I was always just, Mom! Their hugs, giggles, and silly stories were fuel to my fight! They were my biggest motivation to carry on and get out of bed. They made me smile every day and kept some normalcy in a time of chaos. They are what kept me grounded and focused. They inspired me to fight for health, for a longer, better life! They inspired me to grow in character, seek out wisdom and to live for the moments that I could teach them what it means to live abundantly in Christ!

With deep love and gratitude I thank my dedicated and loving husband, Dave. He has seen me at every beautiful high point and at every deep, dark and ugly low point, yet he has never wavered! He has held my hand through it all! He reassured me over and over of his love and of the Lord's constant presence! He has sacrificed time and time again for my happiness, and for the sake of our family, and he does it without complaint! He allowed me to seek help from many without feeling threatened or unappreciated. He was gracious to offer overflowing thanks to all who helped and has always been so willing to help anyone he can! He is generous but asks for very little. Though he is generally serious and intellectual, I love to watch him interact with our children because he is also so silly and playful with them, the jokes and stories go on and on. He is a good Dad and a good role model to our children. I couldn't ask for more than that! Thank you Dave for providing me an exceptional life!

To the one who has given it all. Who has made my life worth anything at all. To my Lord, Father God, His son Jesus Christ and His Holy Spirit. I thank you! And I will continue to thank you for all the days of my life! You are my past, present, and my future. My trust and hope are in you! I thank you, praise you, and give you all the glory!

"Beloved, let us love one another, for love is from God, and whoever loves

has been born of God and knows God."

1 John 4:7

LAURA PENTSA

:INTRODUCTION:
THE REASON I WRITE

Though I am not a theologian, doctor, or even a scholarly trivia genius, through this time of cancer my knowledge certainly increased! I learned about my disease, my body, and my spiritual well being. I gained confidence, knowing that I can share lessons of worth and encouragement with others.

When I was diagnosed with cancer, I searched for a book that would give practical advice and also wisdom from a Godly perspective. I wanted a book that gave attention to all of the layers and aspects of cancer: the physical, mental, & spiritual. I read many good books, but there wasn't that one special book that I felt met everything that I was seeking. My hope and prayer is that this book will.

A book for everyone facing a trial. A book that describes the honest, ugly truths, but also illuminates hope by delivering nourishing, comforting little bits of scripture one small spoonful at a time, one short verse at a time. I want patients to read this and find a friend in me, a fellow patient that has walked this road before, that has learned through the difficulties, and tried to keep a positive and focused eternal perspective. I want the patient's family and friends to gain insight in offering loving support and practical action tips.

I recall feeling weighed down by the burdens of treatment and wondering what my friends who had gone through this might have said. What words of wisdom would they have shared? What advice would they have given? What lessons would they have wanted to leave as a lasting legacy? I'm sad that I couldn't read their books. Maybe in part, that is why I did *not* want to miss this moment and was stirred to begin writing.

Actually putting to paper, the lessons God had lovingly written on my heart during this difficult time.

When I first started writing down these experiences and lessons, I thought I would hide them away and save them for when my children grew up. But as I wrote, the Lord convicted me that others could also benefit from my experiences. I am hopeful that anyone facing a trial can find encouragement and help through the lessons I've learned. My desire is to point them to His Holy Word and to our hope in Christ for comfort, courage, and strength.

I want to share my physical experiences because I sought out other survivors' stories in hopes that I could be prepared, or at the very least, feel normal and not alone. I want to convey my raw emotions because cancer took me on an unexpected rollercoaster with very high peaks and steep, heart-racing drops. I want to tell of those experiences and what helped me remember and hold on to the high points, as well as the things I learned that helped me through the lowest points.

Most of all, I want to pass on the spiritual lessons I've learned, because whether you are a patient or not, these are the real treasures on Earth. The spiritual lessons brought my faith to a very basic, tangible level. Nothing felt theoretical about God; and the horizon of Heaven never felt so close. I hope that I will only grow to know Him more every day of my life, because He is my hope.

This book is a very personal peek into my heart. I desire to be open and real so that you can be honest with yourself and make the most of every single day. This life is so precious and every day is a true gift! May the Lord bless you and keep you!

"The Lord bless you and keep you; the Lord make his face to shine upon you

and be gracious to you; the Lord lift up his countenance upon you

and give you peace." Numbers 6:24-26

Dear Heavenly Father,
We thank you for never leaving us alone. Thank you for hearing our cries and being our peace in times of trial. Please Lord, may anyone struggling today find comfort in you. We ask for your healing hand to be with those who are hurting: physically, mentally, or spiritually. May they cry out to you and draw close. Please be their guide even when there seems to be no way, and help them to know that your Holy Word is a light unto their path. Please give them the courage and strength to carry them through each day. May their faith and trust grow in you Lord. We ask this in the powerful name
of Jesus Christ our Lord and Savior.
Amen

⋮ CHAPTER 1 ⋮
Yesterday, Today and Tomorrow Collide

"Laura, thank you so much for coming in early." The doctor took a moment to pause and drew in a deep breath. He continued, "It turns out that your lump is cancer, and it is aggressive!" My head started to spin. His voice seemed far off, but he went on. "The biopsy shows *it is* actually cancer, and I was surprised. Looking at your ultrasound I didn't expect it to be cancer, but that is the reason we do biopsies." I remember thinking back to the ultrasound-guided biopsy that he had preformed just three days earlier in that very room. Lying there on the exam table and looking at the oval mass on the ultrasound, I was certain I had come in for nothing. It must have been a cyst. I was only being paranoid. But, hearing the doctor say that it was in fact, cancer, seemed unreal. I had *not* been paranoid. I was so glad that I had come in and not ignored the lump!

The doctor opened a thick, stapled packet of printouts and turned to a page full of numbers. He pointed to three zeroes and explained, "You see that the estrogen, progesterone and HER2 receptors are all negative. Zeroes! This tells us about your cancer. It's called triple-negative breast cancer. It is aggressive!" I began to quietly cry. I was in disbelief: shock was crashing through my body and I couldn't stop shaking. My husband tried to calm me by holding my hand, but I could feel his fear too. I looked at him and felt heartbroken knowing that we had to go through this, that I was sick, and that our family had to face this trial. The doctor's words floated through the room and I was desperate to catch them! I was grasping at them trying to listen intently, but my mind was racing! The doctor was still speaking as I scolded myself, "Laura listen! You need to hear what the doctor is saying!" His voice came back into focus." Your markers, the TI67, show that 90% of the cells in your cancer are growing! Normally cells grow at only 15%. One-Five. 15%!" He looked at me, trying to gauge if I understood. He continued, "This means you need to start treatment quickly and you definitely need chemotherapy as a part of your treatment. You will also need surgery and you will have some options with that...." The information kept coming and I hoped this was a nightmare, because I really wanted to wake up.

When the discussion ended, the doctor asked his medical assistant to walk me straight downstairs for the first necessary step towards scheduling treatment. It was the first of a countless number of medical procedures and tests that I would endure as part of my treatment that year.

As the medical assistant guided us there, we passed my mom and kids waiting in the lobby. Mom could see the situation was extremely serious before we even spoke a single word.

That morning had started out perfectly normal. My Mom and I were running errands with my three children who were home on summer break. We were just about to go through the Chick-Fil-A drive thru to grab a quick lunch when my cell phone rang. I remember the call clearly- it was the front office of the breast clinic. They asked me to come in right away, instead of waiting until Monday's scheduled time. The unspoken was more telling than the spoken. I knew this was serious! In a flash, I could already feel the world had flipped upside down. We turned the car around and drove straight to the hospital. Dave met me in the parking lot so we could walk up to the doctor's office together, and my mom lovingly watched our kids in the lobby. How had our lives suddenly changed so drastically?

It was hard to believe that this last thirty minutes had been perfectly normal to the kids and to most everyone else. But for Dave, my mom, and me, time had collided, and what we woke up thinking our life was, now wasn't. The present moment hurt and was overwhelming! That same morning didn't feel like it belonged with that day at all! How was tomorrow ever going to fit with this huge change? Time felt like a giant mess, like a tragic collision.

Once I was seated in the next exam room and my family was all out of sight, the tears began falling. When the next doctor entered the room, she kindly took my hands in hers and said, "I heard that you received some hard news today. Do you have faith?" Her question stunned me! I had not expected this question from a doctor at all, but it was so comforting to look back at her and confidently answer, "Yes, I do have faith!" She held my hands and said, "Good, don't forget that God is with you!" After that, it was straight on to business and she began the physical exam to be sure that my body was ready to begin treatment.

I was still terrified and trembling, facing the start of a very hard year. Her simple question had reminded me though, that I was not alone. I thanked God for bringing me to her that day, and that He gave her the courage to ask me about my faith. It was just the first of many ways the Lord protected and provided for me along this difficult journey of treatment.

"Be strong and courageous.

Do not fear or be in dread of them,

for it is the Lord your God who goes with you.

He will not leave you or forsake you.'"

Deuteronomy 31:6

Below is a timeline showing the first three weeks of my life with cancer.

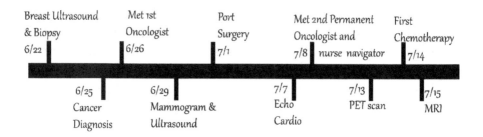

Days later, as the shock transformed into reality, I was able to remember all of the yesterdays of my life. I reflected on the ways that God had always guided our family and comforted us. I was reassured that He would not stop. We would be ok, because yes, "God was with us!"

Allow me to introduce myself the way I would have before cancer:

A Christian. I am very blessed because I felt the Lord speak to my heart back as a teenager and I had devoted myself to Him. He had been my life ever since, and I had sought to live in a way that was obedient to His teachings in the Bible.

A wife. Early in life I prayed that God would provide me with a husband, someone who loved Him more than me and would be a good spiritual example to me. He answered those prayers in Dave. Dave and I had been married for 15 memory-packed years. Dave had been blessed with an incredible understanding of the Bible and was able to teach me things that I may not have easily pieced together without him. He had been faithful and logical while I had been faithful and emotional, so together we made a really good team. We married young, so in many ways we "grew up together" and matured side-by-side. I have been amazed by the way God has shaped and molded Dave. I loved witnessing the boy I married be transformed into a remarkable, admirable man, a man who held my hand and comforted me, even when facing his own fears. He continued to hold my hand and walked into the next hard year of treatment with me, and was devoted and steadfast. I have been so blessed by him!

A mother. This piece of my life didn't come easily. There were many tears and prayers lifted as we waited on the Lord for children. I often wondered if I would ever be called "mother", but with much thankfulness it happened; three times over! They were worth the wait, and perhaps my appreciation for them was expounded because I had dreamed of them for so long.

My son Joel came first after a very complicated, high-risk pregnancy. The Lord was faithful and filled us with His peace throughout the pregnancy. Finally, we were parents and Joel was born. We gave him that name because it meant, "Jehovah is the Lord" and "God is willing". I knew that his name would always remind me that God was willing to allow us to be parents, and for that I've been forever thankful. Joel was a perfect baby, rarely cried and just loved to be held. In fact, he had a bald spot on the back of his head for many months that matched the crook of my elbow because I couldn't bear the idea of putting him down. He grew into an amazing little boy, now age 7. With his inventive, curious, and silly personality, he always kept me on my toes. I loved to hear his ideas and all the funny thoughts that ran through his head. He has taught me so much! A true mama's boy through and through, he would often tell me that he would always be my baby even when he outgrew me, which I expected would happen all too soon!

Then, surprisingly fast right after Joel, came Leah. She was born on an extremely dark, snowy, January day in Cleveland, Ohio but brightened our lives so her "pet name" became Sunshine. It suited her perfectly because her killer smile really did brighten our lives. Leah, now 6, was excelling in school and proved to be a very hard and diligent worker. Creative, talented, responsible, and quiet, she was easy and fun to have around. She was my buddy and we loved all the same hobbies. We tended to always be side by side working on one project or another. Our love for crafting, decorating, shopping, and cooking kept us both messy and happy.

Then there was my adorable baby, Gabrielle. She was already 4, but she had such an innocent and playful spirit that she still seemed even younger. She exuded personality and kindness. She didn't walk - she pranced, twirled, and hopped! She loved to try new things and cuddle. Her giggle was infectious and echoed continuously throughout the house. Kind, thoughtful, and considerate, I loved having our quality alone time when the other two were off at school, and enjoyed the ease of shopping, play-dates, and outings with all of my attention directed on her.

Dave, Joel, Leah, and Gabrielle were the best gifts the Lord had given me here on Earth. I praised Him and thanked Him for their lives. In the days following my diagnosis their faces were what kept me excited about treatment and a cure for cancer. I prayed that the Lord would help me live and continue watching them grow.

Though my life may have looked picture-perfect, nobody's ever really is. We lived a good happy life, but even before cancer, it was not without its own unique struggles. Besides years of infertility struggles, we had also seen other health issues, difficult high-risk pregnancies and deliveries, family issues, drama, as well as my long-lasting struggle with homesickness. You see, Dave was from Ohio while I was from Arizona. When we married, I moved there without hesitation, eager to start our lives together. While his family was large, warm, inviting, passionate, and exciting, I never stopped missing mine or my home church. It was not that I wasn't happy there, because I really was; it was just that somehow, there always was a part of me that hurt. We lived in Ohio for 12 years before moving to Arizona (God's hand was certainly in our move). However, now the roles were reversed. I was home, yet Dave and I still deeply missed his family.

Each of these trials, conflicts, and stages of life were learning experiences. We would hurt and suffer, but we'd also see the Lord's comfort and strength. Each of these were small Ebenezer's to which we could look back and see how God had provided, causing our Faith in Him to grow. Remembering these experiences and that God had been right there all along served as comfort and assurance coming up against cancer.

♡♡♡

After acknowledging that my cancer diagnosis was true, I spent the next year enduring treatment, destroying cancer, and gathering up lessons. I learned more than I could have ever guessed I would. I'd learned about cancer, chemotherapy, surgery, hyperbaric treatments, other people, and a whole lot about myself. But that first day, shaking on the exam table, those were all question marks. A whole heaping pile of question marks! "What does this all mean? Why did this happen? Will the treatment work? What will it feel like? What do I tell my kids? Can I trust this doctor? Do I have any other choices? What do I do next?"

Lots of question marks and the pile of uncertainty just kept piling higher!

> *Tip: When your head is filled with question marks, stop thinking about them or you. Focus on a favorite Bible verse, pray, or sing to the Lord.*

Throughout this book, I will attempt to answer some of those questions, but I also recognize that some questions do not have answers! There are some questions that we cannot dwell on, instead choosing to focus on what we do know.

We do know that God loves us and wants us to focus on Him. When your head is filled with question marks, stop thinking about them or you. Focus on a favorite Bible verse, pray, or sing to the Lord a praise song. Trust me, these Spiritual actions will result in less anxiety and a deeper faith. This does not necessarily come naturally, but the sooner this becomes habit, the sooner you can start to heal emotionally and spiritually from the deep hurt a cancer diagnosis can bring.

"For all who are led by the Spirit of God are sons of God. For you did not receive the spirit of slavery to fall back into fear, but you have received the Spirit of adoption as sons, by whom we cry, "Abba! Father!" The Spirit himself bears witness with our spirit that we are children of God, and if children, then heirs—heirs of God and fellow heirs with Christ, provided we suffer with him in order that we may also be glorified with him."

Romans 8:14-17

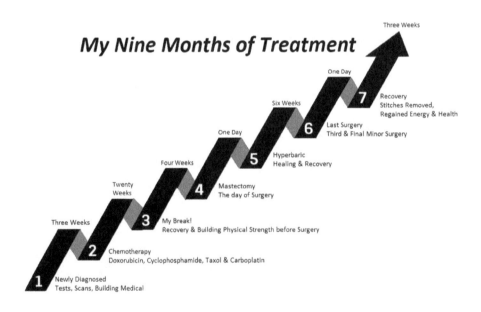

My Nine Months of Treatment

1 — Newly Diagnosed
Tests, Scans, Building Medical

Three Weeks
2 — Chemotherapy
Doxorubicin, Cyclophosphamide, Taxol & Carboplatin

Twenty Weeks
3 — My Break!
Recovery & Building Physical Strength before Surgery

Four Weeks
4 — Mastectomy
The day of Surgery

One Day
5 — Hyperbaric
Healing & Recovery

Six Weeks
6 — Last Surgery
Third & Final Minor Surgery

One Day
7 — Recovery
Stitches Removed, Regained Energy & Health

Three Weeks

Prayer for Spiritual Strength

"For this reason I bow my knees before the Father, from whom every family in heaven and on earth is named, that according to the riches of his glory he may grant you to be strengthened with power through his Spirit in your inner being, so that Christ may dwell in your hearts through faith—that you, being rooted and grounded in love, may have strength to comprehend with all the saints what is the breadth and length and height and depth, and to know the love of Christ that surpasses knowledge, that you may be filled with all the fullness of God. Now to him who is able to do far more abundantly than all that we ask or think, according to the power at work within us, to him be glory in the church and in Christ Jesus throughout all generations, forever and ever. Amen."

Ephesians 3:14-21

i

:CHAPTER 2:
GLEANING WISDOM FROM QUEEN ESTHER

About a month before I was diagnosed with cancer, I had started studying and preparing lesson material for our church's upcoming Fall Women's Retreat, which the Lord convicted me to initiate months earlier. I was really excited about the lesson, but never expected it to become so extremely personal to me. As I've learned, the Lord often provides us with answers and peace through His Word. He used Queen Esther to teach me valuable principles before my fight against cancer.

In chapter four of Esther, Esther realizes that she needs to speak to her husband King Ahasuerus on behalf of the Jews and tell him that Haman, one of the Kings most highly appointed officials, had plotted to destroy the King and annihilate her own people, the Jews. At that time it was not permissible for anyone to approach the King, and to do so was risking possible death. Esther was willing to risk her own life for a chance to save her people. Esther was wise and asked her people, the Jews, for help.

"Then Esther told them to reply to Mordecai, "Go, gather all the Jews to be found in Susa, and hold a fast on my behalf, and do not eat or drink for three days, night or day. I and my young women will also fast as you do. Then I will go to the king, though it is against the law, and if I perish, I perish." Mordecai then went away and did everything as Esther had ordered him." Esther 4:15-17

She asked for help. That was key!

Queen Esther inspired me to do the same, and now I urge you to ask for help, and more specifically prayer support! Having just studied this, I had it on my heart and mind the day I was diagnosed. Part of me wanted to go home, crawl into bed and hide, cry till the tears were all cried out, hope that this nightmare was not real, and wake up back on June 24th, the day before I was diagnosed. None of those ideas would have helped, though. I thank God, because that night was our Ladies Bible Study. I really thought about not going, thinking that maybe I wasn't ready to say anything out loud, and

> *"I needed other people to lift me up in prayer."*

that maybe it would be easier if I just kept it to myself for a few days. No! What did Esther do, before facing this huge, scary life-changing day? She asked her people to pray. That is what I needed, too. I needed others to lift me up in prayer. I was too scared and too weak to even know the words to speak, so I needed the Holy Spirit to intercede for me, and for my fellow believers to lift me up.

"Likewise the Spirit helps us in our weakness. For we do not know what to pray for as we ought, but the Spirit himself intercedes for us with groanings too deep for words." Romans 8:26

I had called and asked my cousins to drive me to Bible Study that night, knowing that I could not. I was weak from emotion, weak from crying, and weak from thinking. Walking into the Ladies Bible Study that night felt like slow-motion. Knowing that our group had just lost a dear friend in recent months to cancer and now asking them to go through it all over again with me was difficult. I didn't want to ask for their help, but I knew it really was what was best. I poured my heart out to them, and they prayed with me. We cried together and read scripture together. It was the first time that day that I was able to breathe. The exhaustion of the day had left me slumped over on the couch, but I was surrounded with love in the comfort of knowing I was not alone.

That night my husband and I held each other and slept. It felt different though. We had changed that day, and our lives would never be the same.

♡♡♡

> **"I was comforted knowing I was not alone."**

A couple days later as we were getting ready for church, we decided to be thankful for the day and take our family picture. Time became very precious. We used this picture later that afternoon on Facebook to ask all of our friends to keep us in prayer. I encourage you to find a way to communicate updates and prayer requests quickly. Some people blog (I didn't know how to do that). Some use Caring Bridge or similar websites set up for this type of communication (this is a great way to go, but having just lost a good friend who used that method, I felt uncomfortable doing something so similar, so soon). Others e-mail or make phone calls. For me, Facebook was the first and easiest method I could think of to get the word out. Most of my friends either saw the posts or were told quickly by mutual friends. I ended up needing my sister-in-law to copy my posts and send an e-mail out to our "Non-Facebook" family and that worked well, so that everyone knew exactly what was going on.

I will include many of my Facebook posts in this book as a way to show you my specific thoughts and memories while I was still in the heat of battle. The following was my first public post regarding cancer.

Facebook Post:
June 28th

Calling out to all my prayer warrior friends & family! This Thursday I (Laura) was diagnosed with Triple-Negative, Stage 2 Breast Cancer. It is an aggressive cancer, but we are hopeful

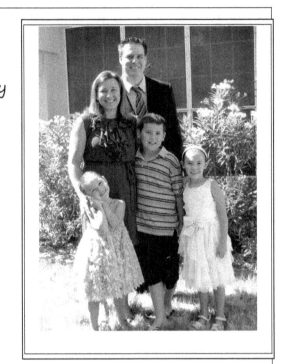

that it will be beat! Please keep my family in your prayers! Specifically, please pray that tomorrow's mammogram and Dr apt go well and that they confirm that there is only one mass. I will keep you all posted, and please feel free to share this with anyone who prays! I've seen God working in my life in so many ways over the years and I know He is with me now and knows my need.

"Be strong and of good courage, do not fear nor be afraid of them; for the Lord your God, He is the One who goes with you. He will not leave you nor forsake you." Deuteronomy 31:6

The second lesson I learned from Queen Esther was that the Lord can use the "bad" things in our life to create something new and beautiful. I prayed that the Lord would somehow use my cancer for something good. I knew that I might never see that transformation, but I knew that I could ask the Lord to use this for His purpose and to His glory. It had already triggered a transformation because it gave me a new sense of purpose.

When I thought about all the bad things that happened in Queen Esther's life and seeing how God used her in such an inspiring way, I knew He could do the same for me. Maybe I wouldn't save an entire nation, but if I could help someone in some way, then I was happy for that.

Let's look at some of the hardships from the book of Esther for a moment and think about how the Lord used those situations to provide abundantly and make something new. Below shows Queen Esther's "lemons," or tragedies, and how the Lord used them.

❖ Esther's parents die - Mordecai raises Esther.
❖ The women are taken from their homes - Esther is placed in the King's palace where she could be used.
❖ Mordecai overhears a death plot - The King's life is saved.
❖ Esther asks the Jews to fast and pray for her - The King hears Esther and finds favor in her.
❖ The King can't sleep - He reads the history book, reading the exact passage needed to remind him of an unpaid reward to Mordecai.
❖ Haman makes an exact plan to exterminate the Jews - The plan is exactly reversed to make the intended victims now become the victors!

Seeing what Esther was up against helped keep my battle in perspective. If the Lord can orchestrate all of that in Esther's life, why should I doubt that He can use my hardship for something better?

❖ Laura's Cancer -_____

Just wondering how this might be used and knowing that there were unlimited ways the Lord could fill in the blank, made me feel like this diagnosis was not a waste. It gave me a sense of purpose and value. At times, I even felt like I was on an untold, secret mission just waiting for my orders.

"And who knows whether you have not come to the kingdom for such a time as this?" Has the Lord been preparing you for such a time as this? Had He been preparing me all along?

"Then Mordecai told them to reply to Esther, "Do not think to yourself that in the king's palace you will escape any more than all the other Jews. For if you keep silent at this time, relief and deliverance will rise for the Jews from another place, but you and your father's house will perish. And who knows whether you have not come to the kingdom for such a time as this?"

Esther 4:13-14

> **The Lord can use the "bad" things in our life to create something beautiful.**

About eight weeks into treatment, I was blessed to go and present the lesson on Queen Esther at the Fall Women's Retreat. That lesson and these women are so dear to my heart! Here is a picture of our group holding up a lesson poster from the weekend. The yellow tulips began as cut-outs of lemons. As we discussed each of Esther's "lemons", the trials in her life, and the way God changed those into something new and beautiful, we placed the lemons into this beautiful tulip arrangement, illustrating how God can make all things new!

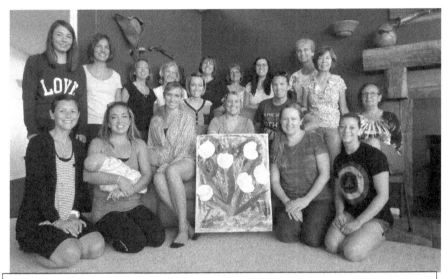

August 24th

Had an amazing time at our women's retreat! Great friends, fun projects and an inspiring lesson about Queen Esther. I started planning for this lesson just before I was diagnosed and I believe that God was preparing my heart, so that I can trust that God will be glorified even in this difficult time.

:CHAPTER 3:
HAIR TODAY, GONE TOMORROW

A whole chapter about hair? Yes, a whole chapter! Some cancer patients do not lose their hair, but for many this is a common side effect of chemotherapy. I thought I'd share a detailed look at my own experience so that others can perhaps be better prepared for what may happen or what can help make the experience a bit less upsetting.

The Wig

First of all, be sure to find out which chemotherapy medication your oncologist will be administering and if hair loss is likely. If the answer is yes, I would suggest getting prepared. Start by asking your oncologist for a prescription for a "cranial prosthesis". This is technical jargon for a wig! It must be written up this way for insurance to help pay for the wig. Also, ask for a recommendation or a list of places to go to purchase one. Although many places sell wigs, your insurance may not be accepted at all of them. It is also very helpful to go somewhere that often works with cancer patients. If insurance still will not assist with the cost, seek out help from local non-profit organizations.

Coincidentally, 1 year post treatment, I became involved in helping support our Phoenix area non-profit organization, "Don't Be A Chump! Check for a Lump!" One of our main missions is to assist breast cancer patients with free wigs when insurance is not available. A wig is so much more than just hair; it really can aid with comfort, confidence, and a sense of identity.

I scheduled an appointment at our closest shop. They got me in very quickly and I took my husband along for much-needed support. At first, when I walked in all of the "hair dressers" were busy so I just started looking around. I found a wig with long beautiful hair. It was similar in color to my own, but a bit longer and I imagined it would look quite pretty, maybe even better than my own hair. As I pondered those long locks, one of the kind sales ladies approached me to help. I told her that I was there for an appointment and that because of chemo, I expected to start losing my hair in the next few weeks. She saw the wig I was looking at and said, "Oh, honey, if you'd like to try this one on, we can... but I really think you'll want one with short hair." She had a kind face and I tended to believe that she meant well, but I also thought, "Well, that's kind of gutsy, how can she be so presumptuous to even guess that she knows what I want? She doesn't even know me." So we sat down, and she pulled the long beautiful wig over my full head of hair. It looked awful and it felt even worse! At this point, I got it... okay, she may not know me, but she does know wigs! It was time for me to trust her. She went on to explain how hot wigs can feel, especially in Phoenix, Arizona. She also explained how the hair will not feel just like my own and on delicate tender "chemo skin" the hair can feel really rough and itchy. Finally a point that really hit home was, "Your hair will come back, but it will be very short, it might be nice to get used to yourself looking a bit different, because things are going to change." All really good points! It was still extremely hard to digest or accept being only a few days into this new diagnosis.

However, I knew she was right. It pained me to know that this was all really about to happen. I remember feeling a bit silly as we tried on several wigs. She tried to help me visualize what it would look like without my own hair beneath it, but it was hard to really imagine. It felt like dress up, not like something I would seriously have to wear publicly and feel normal about! She was also very glad I came in before my hair had actually fallen out, because they were able to special order the wig with shades of hair that most closely resembled my natural color. Later on, this really did make the wig feel more "me". I did end up choosing a wig that day and, it was just above my shoulders and did end up looking very pretty and very natural. Below (left) is a picture I took about a month before I was diagnosed, with my own hair. On the right is a picture with my brand new wig.

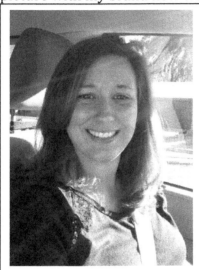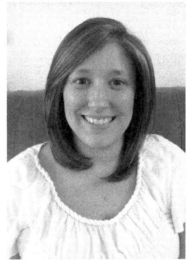

The same day I purchased the wig, the kind "hair dresser" also convinced me to buy several head wraps to have ready at home. That was really difficult for me. Trying to imagine these head wraps as if they were going to be my new "normal," I didn't really know if I'd even be comfortable using them. Would my kids pull at them? Would I feel weird wearing them? Would I be able to tie them on properly without help? How would I ever do this at home without the encouraging "hair dressers" boosting my confidence?

Still, I bought them. I chose colors that I liked and knew would go well with my clothes. It was a really hard day, but the staff at that shop really helped. My husband hugged me when I needed it and told me I would still be beautiful when I didn't really believe it myself.

A Hair Cut

I was told that my hair would start falling out around Day 14 after my first dose of chemotherapy, so I made an appointment to get a short pixie haircut on Day 10. I had read that having short hair before it starts to fall out makes the experience a little easier, so I started looking up pixie cuts online. I would have NEVER tried a pixie cut, never even considered it, but since this was a time for change, I might as well try one out that I thought looked cute.

I really thought about whether my kids should be there with me and I decided they were at an age where it could benefit them to be a part of this small step. So, I used that morning to really explain the medicine to my kids. I explained how this medicine was going to help save mommy's life, and kill those yucky cancer cells; but sometimes that very helpful medicine will do some things that I don't like, too - things like make me tired, make me feel yucky, and even make my hair fall out. I tried to answer all of their questions with the positive answer: "It will all be worth it". "The medicine will help us get rid of the cancer". "The medicine will help Mommy to get healthy". I also, explained getting this hair cut would help me not feel so upset when it started coming out and, that it would not be as messy and could be something fun to try since I wouldn't have to mind it for too long anyhow. My kids were amazing, and they did really great with all of that information and wanted to be there to see me get my long hair get cut super short!

I took the kids and my mom along to the hair cut. I chose to go to a close friend named Megan, who is also a great hairstylist. I showed her a picture on my phone of the actress Anne Hathaway, and asked her to make it happen. Megan was amazing and took long strands and snipped them carefully away so that we'd have a good length to donate for someone else needing a wig. We explained to the kids how donating hair worked and that helped them feel good, knowing that my hair would be helping someone else. She snipped and cut and we actually managed to smile and even giggle through the appointment. I think having the kids there helped me look at the positive and not get upset. While I was putting on a brave face, in part, by the end I think I had even convinced myself that this wasn't really a bad day at all. When we were done, I was surprised how different I looked, and even more surprised that I did, kind-of even like it! In fact, it made me feel brave; it was like I looked in the mirror at someone preparing for battle. I was ready to fight and my new hair felt like a physical preparation for that battle. I could feel my attitude changing and preparing for what was to come, and I thanked the Lord for my courage and asked Him to keep it coming!

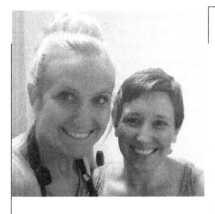

July 21st

Thank you Megan for making a very difficult transition into something special, and bringing me smiles. I never would have picked short hair or a bald head, and I can't say that I'm super happy about it. However; I know this is just hair and that the people that care about me are not going to care one bit about what my head looks like. Even more I am so thankful that I don't have to worry about feeling rejected by my husband who has loved me on the best and worst of days for the past 15 years. He sees me for my heart, just as the Lord does. Thank you God for Dave!

1 Samuel 16:7b ESV "For the Lord sees not as man sees: man looks on the outward appearance, but the Lord looks on the heart."

The next day, my husband took me out for a Date Night. I wanted him to take out this "new" girl and for us to just enjoy each other before the hair was gone and the chemotherapy effects started to take over my body. It was a bitter sweet evening. It felt like the end of a chapter. I was unsure what the new chapter would hold, but I was thankful I was not going into it alone.

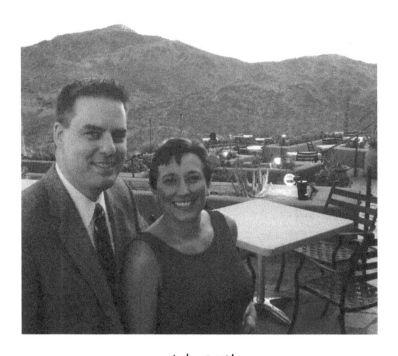

July 25th

Had a wonderful date night at

Different Pointe of View!

Losing My Hair

I had enjoyed a few short days of the new pixie cut. It was almost enough to start recognizing myself in the mirror again, but it was just long enough to start mentally preparing for the hair to actually begin falling out. Here is a big tip!!! Before your hair starts to fall out, get a drain cover. (I've since seen them at dollar stores.) That is something I did not know to buy. It would have helped!

My chemo nurse Jen had told me that around Day 14, I would probably begin losing my hair. She was very right. On Day 14, I went with my cousin and friend Marie to my second dose of AC chemotherapy. That morning, I was still feeling quite proud of my new pixie cut, and my head was full of hair. Nothing seemed to be different that morning. In fact, I had even wondered... what if I am one

Tip: Get a drain cover for the shower!!!

of the few that can take this medicine and not lose their hair? What if this hair cut didn't need to happen? Hmmm... well... that evening, my head started to ache.

It was like a dull ache, much like when I was little girl and my mom had braided my hair a little too tightly, only to find at the end of the day that you take out that braid and your head feels sore. Well, it felt exactly like that, but the soreness didn't go away after a couple minutes. I knew my hair was going to start falling out. The next day, it began. I woke up to a few strands of hair on my pillow, and then quite a few came out when I combed my hair, followed by a good handful coming out in the shower.. Ok.. it is really happening. I got obsessed. Honestly, all day I only thought about hair! "How many days will this happen? Am I going to be like our pet bunny who sheds for weeks each season and gets the entire house dusty with fur? Will my scalp hurt worse than this?" Well, the answer came quiet surprisingly the next morning. I woke with a very full head of hair, and only a bit of hair left on the pillow, but then I went to take my shower.

It was Day 16 now and my scalp was very tender, and when the warm water hit my scalp, something I did not expect happened. It all started coming out! More than handfuls! More than clumps! It was like my pores just opened up and released the hairs from my head. I was scared! I felt like I might suffocate or drown from the never ending hairs flowing from my head over my face and body. My shower floor was covered and, my drain was clogged. I grabbed a washcloth and tried to uncover the drain. I put the wash cloth above it to prevent the hair from going down. I wish I'd bought a drain cover! Why didn't anyone tell me that this was not just a few weeks of hair thinning, but a very sudden, very dramatic event?

It was not a good morning! I cried and the hair kept flowing. I eventually got the shower floor cleaned up and flopped down on my bed and I prayed for the Lord to cast out my fear. I cried and I prayed until the tears stopped. When I had calmed, I went and got out my head wrap, ripped off the tags and put it on my head. I looked at the mirror, and it felt like I was looking at a stranger. The yellow sick skin had started from chemo, the red puffy eyes from crying, and the soft pink wrap

> **"Don't give up,
> keep fighting!"**

was on my head. Who was this person? It was still me, and over the next few days I would come to recognize that, but Day 16 was not that day.

I don't give all this detail for the sake of sympathy or to scare new patients. I tell this so that you can know what to expect. Prepare yourself and remember that even if it is a bad day, the next can be better. Don't give up, keep fighting, and keep getting stronger. When you are weak the Lord is strong. Let Him hold you up and care for you.

> *"Are not five sparrows sold for two pennies? And not one of them is*
>
> *forgotten before God. Why, even the hairs of your head are all numbered.*
>
> *Fear not; you are of more value than many sparrows." Luke 12: 6-7*

By the following week, I had gotten fairly used to my new head wraps, and I had even worn my wig to church, but there were still a few strands of hair that never came out. It was really weird-looking. I wouldn't let anyone see me without something covering my head. To me, I looked like that awful creature, Gollum, from the Lord of the Rings Movies. Though I'm not a huge fan of those movies, that is all I could think of when it came to these last few strands of hair, so I called on my Dad for help.

He was the perfect person to help me with this. He has been shaving his head for years and keeps his head smooth or with a very minimal buzz cut. He kept encouraging me that I was going to love being bald. He had sent me pictures of beautiful brave cancer survivors who modeled with their bald heads, and he knew I could do it too. So I asked him to come finish what the medicine had started. We went out in my backyard and he used the electric clippers to shave off those last few pesky strands. He left me the clippers in case they grew back. They didn't... well at least not until all of my hair started growing back about 5 months later.

Calling on Dad for help was a good decision. He and I will never forget that experience, and I don't think anyone else could have been so supportive that day. Sometimes it is the strangest things that bring people even closer together.

My shining bald head was much easier for me to accept and I did end up being very comfortable at home. My kids loved to rub it, and strangely, even kiss it. I never loved my bald head, but it did eventually feel normal.

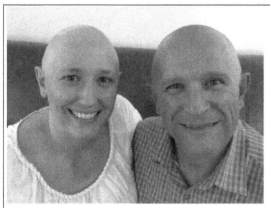

Sept 23rd
Never wanted to look THIS much like my Dad, (but at least he's good looking)
This picture was taken almost 2 months ago, and I am finally feeling brave enough to share it. My Dad has been encouraging me to be bold, brave and beautiful and

to embrace the bald. I can't say I've done great on that last part, but I'm getting there. Not many Dads could handle shaving off those last miserable Gollum-like hairs, but he did, and I'm grateful for all the ways he has been showing love.

Eyebrows & Eyelashes

My eyebrows and eyelashes did all fall out, but very slowly. It took months before all of them had fallen out. I could tell it was happening as they thinned, so I really tried to memorize where my eyebrows started and stopped. I used brown eye shadow and an angled makeup brush to fill them in. Eventually, I learned just how to mimic the shape so that by the time they were gone, nobody could even tell that it was only makeup.

I never attempted anything for the lashes, it just wasn't worth it to me. But I did hear some ladies say they used false lashes. My eyes felt dry from the chemo so I didn't want to bother them. For instructions on how to apply eyebrow makeup, YouTube has many videos dedicated the topic. Eyebrows, a little bronzer and some lip gloss helped me feel "normal". Sometimes it's the little things.

Though I did wear my wig to church, special events, nicer restaurants and the kids' school programs, I generally felt uncomfortable in it. It was hot and scratchy, plus my kids always wanted to touch it, which terrified me, fearing they would pull it off. Plus, people who know you are wearing a wig tend to study you and want to touch it. Though it wasn't my favorite thing to wear, I was incredibly thankful to have it as an option. It was amazing to feel "normal" when I wore it. I felt like I could blend in with a crowd and not look like a sick patient. I liked that I could still wear something fancy and not have an awkward scarf ruin the look for special events. It helped me feel like a beautiful woman and it boosted my confidence.

For my day-to-day activities, scarves were the most comfortable. Again, YouTube shows a variety of ways to tie them. I was able to find very inexpensive scarves or borrow some. This way, I could match them to my clothes and it made it a little bit more fun. The chemo head wraps were easier, and some were very soft. I liked having a couple for sleeping and wearing once in a while, but if I were to do it all over, I'd do mostly scarves and save my money.

Looking back, I also learned that losing your hair can be a blessing. HOW? Most people see your head wrap or scarf and realize that you are battling cancer. Most people knew someone who had been on this journey and they were generally more considerate. Good conversations often happened simply because people could tell I was sick. Many people face extreme illness but don't have an obvious physical signal to tell people what's going on. I was eventually thankful that my scarves became a signal to people, and it made discussing my disease much easier.

Oddly, being bald made me more confident overall. Though I never liked being bald, I realized that I had given my hair, makeup, and clothing too much credit. My friends and family liked me for me. They really didn't care about the rest. Knowing this fueled my confidence.

"Charm is deceitful, and beauty is vain, but a woman who fears the Lord is to be praised." Proverbs 31:30

Hair Growing Back

My hair began to start growing back toward the end of my chemotherapy. I was on different medications and was surprised that by my last chemo, my whole head had a small short layer of fuzz. The tips were almost invisible/white. Once my hair was about 1/2 inch long, I had the white tips cut off.

Megan called it a "dusting", just the very little tips being trimmed off so it looked a bit darker.

My hair came in a slightly darker-brown color. I have a few more grays than before, and the most drastic change was that it came in very, very curly! I only had a couple very minimal trims to help the shape, and within the first year after chemotherapy it grew 4" long.

When it first started growing back, I felt like I could watch it getting longer everyday. It was thrilling! I thought it looked full before it actually did. I would send pictures to family trying to show my new hair, but I'd have to get the lighting just right or you couldn't even see it. It felt strange when people eventually just thought I liked to wear my hair short. I thought it was so obvious to everyone what I'd been through, but to most people, I just looked like a normal, healthy girl with very short hair. That is a good thing, too.

Often, I now find it strange that I need to reintroduce myself to acquaintances. For example, other moms at school often don't even recognize me, having gone from the mom with golden brown hair, to the one with the scarf, to the one with dark short curls. It is sometimes a little awkward, but I usually find that if I just initiate the conversation with, "Hi, I'm Laura... we worked in so-and-so's class last year on the holiday party... I know I look quite different now, but I'm feeling good and like my new curls." ... usually, people sigh with relief that they don't have to wonder if that's you or they now realize who you are and things are just much easier.

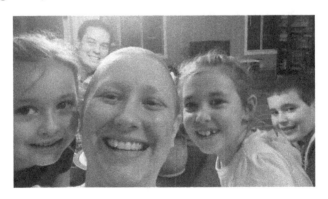

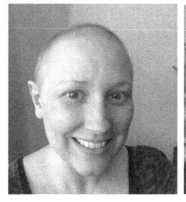 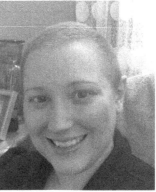

Above: Last week of chemo   Above: 1 month after chemo

Below: 3 months after chemo   Below: 4 months after chemo

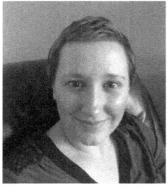 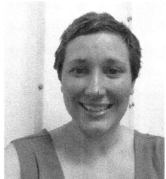

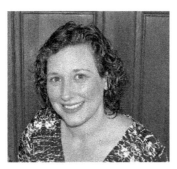

One year after Chemo.

I loved watching my hair grow!

:CHAPTER 4:
BUILDING A TEAM

After I was diagnosed, it felt like a tornado swept me up, turned over my life, and dropped me and my date book permanently in the doctor's office. I remember the first two weeks being just packed with appointments and tests. It was confusing and overwhelming! My advice is to ask all of your questions, seek out extra help for getting organized, and request reinforcements.

What compounded this entire timeframe for us was that my husband Dave had accepted a new job only days prior to my diagnosis, which meant changing to a new hospital network and employer. This made for some unique complexities, such as switching insurance and waiting for our new id numbers and cards to be assigned. Switching doctors after just starting this cancer journey caused much confusion regarding medical bills for the first few months. It was certainly a unique set of circumstances. In hindsight, it really was all for the best because I loved my new medical team!

Building a Medical Team

I think the most important character trait in an oncologist is someone you feel confidence in and comfortable asking questions to. When I had to seek out an oncologist on my new medical insurance, I felt at a complete loss! We received a list of about 60 oncologists to choose from. The list showed their name, specialty, and contact information. There was nothing personal to it, and I remember crying in front of my computer screen thinking, "Do I really have to Google every single name on this list and make a guess as to who would be best for me?"

It just seemed like a gigantic mountain in the way! I wanted to start treatment right away, not spend days researching doctors.

Well, a few beautiful things happened that day. Melaney, a wonderful friend of mine, stopped by to spend a little time with my kids, and she was like an angel that day. She was a nurse, and though she did not work in oncology, she did do some training at the breast surgery center where my new care team would be. She was able to calm me and reassure me

> *Tip: Please, ask people for help along the way, you cannot do this all by yourself!*

that I would be in great hands, that the team there was fantastic, and that the nurses had been outstanding. She said she would have recommended this hospital to me or her own family. Wow! That took a huge burden off my shoulders. The stress from the list just shrunk from Mount Everest down to about Camelback Mountain, which is still considered an extremely difficult and dangerous hike here in Arizona!

Then Dave called and told me that he had sent out an e-mail to his colleagues at the new hospital and asked if anyone had personal experiences with oncologists whom they would highly recommend. Suddenly our list was narrowed down to three! Boom, that mountain was gone! Thank You, Lord for all the people you have put on our path that have shown us kindness and love. Even through these recommendations, people have given us so much help!

"Trust in the Lord with all your heart,

and do not lean on your own understanding.

In all your ways acknowledge him,

and he will make straight your paths." Proverbs 3:5-6

At this point I was down to three names. I prayed and asked the Lord to let me have peace about one of them, and that they would have space to quickly accept a new patient. I started to search their names and though any of the three may have been great, there was one that stood out to me. In an interview I watched on-line, the doctor basically quoted the golden rule, explaining that it was the way he approached his medical practice. That gave me the peace I needed to make my choice. I called his office and made an appointment for the very next day! This was an answered prayer. The Lord eased my anxieties and lifted that burden. I had found my oncologist! Within 24 hours I was in his office and he had a plan of action ready for me to begin treatment.

"Peace I leave with you; my peace I give to you. Not as the world gives do I give to you. Let not your hearts be troubled, neither let them be afraid."

John 14:27

I believe it is critical to trust your doctor because having cancer is scary and there are so many unknowns. However, when you trust your doctor, you can let them work out the details of what your body physically needs and plan accordingly. That

> *Tip: Starting with your diagnosis, keep all records and scans in a file or folder so you can easily take them to appointments.*

way, you can focus on the rest of what really matters: getting well and spending time with loved ones. Once you have your oncologist, they will be helpful in building the rest of your medical team. For me, I chose several other members of my team based on his suggestions.

The second person you want to add to your team is an Oncology Nurse Navigator. This person has served as an oncology nurse and knows the ins-and-outs of cancer treatment. This person can assist in navigating healthcare, and is someone you can turn to if you don't know what will happen next or need more contacts. They are terrific at sifting through the huge pile of question marks. As my Oncology Nurse Navigator, Dawn had so many resources to provide. She walked me through the medical terminology that accompanied my specific diagnosis, and she provided me an organizational method for my medical records, labs, and contacts. She supplied me with the paperwork for my medical directives and presented me with information on support groups, classes, and showed me a medical library I was able to access. She referred me and introduced me to a nutritional counselor and the clinical exercise specialist. She also offered contact information for genetic testing and possible clinical trials. Though I did not pursue the clinical trials, I was thankful to know they were available.

She also gave me a great piece of advice, warning me to resist the urge to Google and to only use the websites she or my doctors recommended because the internet has unlimited tales of worst case scenarios and negativity. Both would have been incredibly dangerous for me at that point.

Overall, this oncology navigator is extremely helpful and has valuable information. I met with her a handful of times throughout treatment and she efficiently navigated my medical path through treatment.

The third person I suggest you getting to know is a nutritional counselor. I actually sought help from two sources: a family friend, Mike, who is both a chiropractor and nutrition expert. As well as the hospitals Oncology Dietitian, Terry, who I had

If you are looking for nutritional advice, I've included many tips in Chapters 6 and 12.

been introduced and referred to by my Oncology Navigator. Nutrition is an extremely important part of cancer therapy and recovery! Nutritional counselors can provide specific nutritional guidance during your cancer journey and help to adjust when side effects or physical ailments occur. I met with them a total of four times and the information was extremely valuable. I was taught how to eat during chemotherapy to keep strong and battle some of the side effects. We spoke again presurgery with a focus on getting my immune system up and strong. We also met post-surgery for a long-lasting lifestyle approach to stay well and help lower my risks of reoccurrence. I've met many patients who did not meet with any nutritional counselors and while it was optional for me, I believe their advice still remains vital and I very highly recommend it!

Having three children, I also chose to seek genetic counseling. The genetic test did not show any genetic mutations at this time which means the test was not conclusive on the cause being genetic or environmental. Even though I am left not fully understanding how or why I had cancer, I was still glad to have the information. If the test had shown a genetic mutation, that information could have helped my doctors watch closely for other cancers that pose a high risk and would be a warning for my children, too. This was not my takeaway and there is some comfort in that, also. The genetic counselor was kind and supportive while explaining what each result may mean and how that information was useful to our situation. I found this experience very emotional.

> *Tip: Treat the nurses and medical staff as part of your team! You won't regret it!*

Even though you do not get to choose nurses and other medical support, I want to emphasize that they are important! They are on the team. They are the hands that administer medicine, the hands that position you for tests, and the voices that talk you through a phone call. In short, they are the care team! Treat them that way; like you are all on one team! Be helpful to them, tell them everything they need to know about your health, be patient, be respectful, be polite, and be kind. These people are often a wealth of knowledge, too. They know how to help with many side effects. They care about your comfort and they have chosen their profession because they are intelligent and compassionate.

The Medical Team Checklist:

Doctors:
- ☐ Oncologist (First!): Treats cancer
- ☐ Oncology Surgeon: Removes cancer surgically
- ☐ Reconstructive Surgeon: Provides cosmetic reconstruction surgeries
- ☐ Radiologist: Uses X-ray and radiation to treat cancer

Other Medical Support:
- ☐ Oncology Nurse Navigator: Provides information and contacts
- ☐ Clinical Trials: May have new treatments available
- ☐ Nutritional Counselor: Provides information on how to boost your health through good nutrition for each stage of treatment
- ☐ Cancer Genetic Risk Assessment: Assess or genetically test to determine the likelihood of finding a hereditary or environmental cancer condition
- ☐ Social Work: Financial and legal assistance

The Support Team Checklist:

☐ Prayer Team: Anyone and everyone who will pray
☐ Emotional Support Team: Your spouse, parents, family, friends. Have a few, because this is draining and exhausting for them, too!
☐ A Cancer Survivor: Someone who has walked this road or is living with cancer
☐ Appointment Companion: People to take you to appointments, possibly take notes and be your support
☐ The Organizer: Someone to organize your helpers and communicate your needs
☐ Helpers: People who are willing to help, whatever the need is
☐ The Communicator: Someone to forward updates to everyone
☐ Other _____

"A joyful heart is good medicine,

but a crushed spirit dries up the bones." Proverbs 17:22

Building A Support Team

Having cancer affects each patient differently, but it is safe to say you will need support. Though each person may have different needs based on their home, family, or health, it is a good idea to ask a few people to help in *specific* ways early on. You can always change things later based on your preferences or needs.

> **Tip: Prayer warriors are precious, but remember that you need to be on that team too! Keep praying for yourself and others!**

I was told by many professionals that I had an outstanding support team. It was true! I attribute this to a couple things. First, I am surrounded with a lot of truly beautiful, faithful Christians. Our family and church family all serve the Lord and are eager and willing workers. The love they extended was like watching the Lord's hands work right in front of me. Their extension of His love reminds me of these wonderful verses:

"Abide in me, and I in you. As the branch cannot bear fruit by itself, unless it abides in the vine, neither can you, unless you abide in me. I am the vine; you are the branches. Whoever abides in me and I in him, he it is that bears much fruit, for apart from me you can do nothing. If anyone does not abide in me he is thrown away like a branch and withers; and the branches are gathered, thrown into the fire, and burned." John 15:4-6

Second, if someone offered to help, I took them up on it. I think many times people miss out on help because they don't accept it. I sometimes struggled with this too, thinking that I didn't want to be a burden, or not knowing what task or responsibility I would even have for them (off the top of my head). I thought back to the times that I had helped someone who was sick or just had a new baby and how happy that service made me. I believe that allowing people to help me was a part of the reason that I had such an amazing support structure, and I also know it was good for the people who care about me, too. If someone offered help, I tried to always respond with: "Well, if you're sure that you really don't mind, then I'm certain we could use your help. My aunt is helping me organize those needs. Can I give her your information or would you like to call her?" I will dive more into that soon, but basically that allowed the person an opportunity to sign up for a responsibility that they felt comfortable doing and it spread the need out so nobody (except Dave & Mom) felt overworked or overburdened.

Along with physical support, Queen Esther really showed me early on that I needed prayer support, and for me that was critical. I felt so much comfort and strength knowing

> *Tip: Accept offers of help! And find someone to help organize that help!*

throughout the day or during tests, that others had me covered with prayer. It is hard to describe, but once you experience it, you'll be so glad you asked for their support. This is also a wonderful way for people to help. It is something they can do anytime, anywhere! I would get texts throughout the day saying something simple like, "just prayed for you" or "was just thinking of you, do you have any specific prayer requests?" I loved those messages. It was so encouraging and I knew I was loved and cared for. Ask for prayer! Also, don't forget to pray yourself. You are on that team too, so pray for your own needs and theirs too!

Your spouse, family, and friends can be a great source of emotional support. I found that there are some people I could openly share medical information with and others who I can cry with, lending a sympathetic ear, while perhaps someone else is that special person who made me laugh no matter how rotten the moment felt. I tried to surround myself with people that cared. I learned to lean on them for support, and also tried to remember that seeing me sick was really hard on them.

They were going through their own stresses and sometimes needed to lean on me for support from time to time as well. For some friends this can be emotionally overwhelming and exhausting, so it is nice to have more than just one person to share these struggles with. Since some of the same people often end up covering many of the day-to-day responsibilities, this can also cause them extra fatigue and stress as well. I know my husband Dave really stepped up and got up early to get the kids ready for school, learned to do the girls' hair, and checked their backpacks. He often bore the bedtime responsibilities all on his own, and that was a change as I'd always been there to do things for our children. My mom also pitched in with the kids, the mountains of laundry, and the cleaning. All of those stresses are hard on the family. They were my go-to for support, but I still had to remember that they needed support too!

Sometimes, someone you were not very close to can become a person who really comes through and supports you. I grew up knowing one of my mom's lifelong friends Esther, and in recent years we really had not spent tons of time together. But because of her own life experiences, she knew how to be an outstanding encourager! She had lived through trials and seen family members battle cancer. Those experiences created a beautiful talent which she graced me with. She was a consistent source of encouragement and was extremely special to me. Even people you might not expect to be a big part of your journey might become extremely precious to you.

If you don't feel like your needs are being met, ask your nurse navigator or oncologist for a list of cancer support groups. There are many groups set up for this very purpose; other patients and survivors want to be there for each other and this can be a really wonderful way to talk through things and find comfort and support.

I found it so encouraging and helpful to talk with other survivors. At first I didn't know anyone that had my same diagnosis, but within weeks a mutual friend had given me information on someone who survived my exact diagnosis and had had very similar treatment. I e-mailed with her a few times and found so much comfort in knowing that she had made it through the treatment and was living a healthy life. Now, being a 1 year survivor myself, I have had opportunities to help others just starting their fight against cancer. I love to offer my support and advice, which is very common among survivors, so reach out to survivors and you will both benefit. If you don't know anyone with a similar diagnosis, a support group may be of help.

I did not like going to any appointments by myself. While some of the patients I saw did everything on their own and preferred it that way, I did not. My mom came with me to most of my tests and while I could have often gone by myself, I think nervousness and boredom would have set in while I waited. With Mom there, we always had something to chat about. If I did get nervous, she could help me relax. She was a second set of ears, and sometimes asked just the right question that I would have missed. Plus, sometimes I was quite tired after an appointment and I could rest on the drive home. When Mom was not able to come, either my husband or a friend would come to keep me company. For me, having a companion at appointments helped keep me cheerful and at ease. Plus, it gave us some great quality time, which is also very important.

> *Tip: Survivors often like to help others going through treatment. And support groups are another source for comfort and help.*

"As for you, brothers, do not grow weary in doing good."

2 Thessalonians 3:13

> Sept 4th Out to breakfast with my amazing mom after morning blood work. She has been at my side every step of the way! Love you Mom!

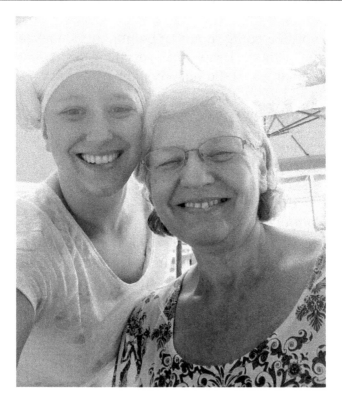

One of the most difficult parts of asking for support and help is to organize and orchestrate that help. Many times, I could have just said, "Never mind, I don't want any help", because it seemed like too many phone calls and too much trouble. It can be awkward to ask for specific help at times, but thankfully I have an incredibly kind, intelligent, organized, polite aunt who was willing to help me with all of that! She became my support team organizer, and I do not know what I would have done without my Aunt Corinne! When my side effects really started to impact my daily living, my aunt and I came up with a specific list of ways people could help if they offered. So whenever someone would say, "What can I do to help?" we could ask which area they'd be able to help in or I'd just give them my aunt's e-mail!

This brings me to all of the helpers. I was truly blessed because there were many people who wanted to help our family. I did not want to overburden anyone, so my aunt did a wonderful job of rotating and organizing who would help and when. We came up with three basic categories of helpers: childcare, food, and appointments. As people offered to help she would find out how they could help in those areas and it really worked out well for our family. I also had a couple people with ongoing specific jobs, like my brother Steve who lent Dave a hand with home improvement projects and my friend Stephanie who came weekly to work with our kids to make sure homework packets got finished and turned in.

Below is an example of how we categorized our families needs:

Food	Babysitters	Housework	Other
Cut and prep fruits & veggies	Watch the kids for appointments	Light Cleaning	Transportation to Doctor Appointments
Bring a hot prepared meal	Take the kids out for a fun activity	Laundry or Ironing	Stay with Laura at appointments
Specific shopping needs	Come and swim with the kids	Organizing and Dishes	Run Errands (ex: Dry Cleaning)

Last, but certainly not least, was the communicator. Within a day of my diagnosis, I knew something needed to change. My phone was dinging with texts and voicemails all the time. I wanted to tell everyone what was going on, but it was emotional and exhausting! It was like a full-time job. That is when I decided that I needed to type up a basic public update as things happened and post it to Facebook. My lovable sister-in-law Adrienne would copy that exact post and e-mail or text it out to anyone else that should receive an update. This may not be the perfect method, but I would encourage you to find a system that works for you and your loved ones so that you can get information out quickly to everyone. It took so much pressure off of me and I didn't have to worry about communications. Everyone was getting the same information at the same time. It was really helpful to have her forwarding out information.

With your specific needs, think about who can help you and how you can make it work for your family. Help should be helpful, not stressful! Remember that you can make requests and change them as treatment goes on. If people can help, be grateful when it works out, but also remember that this is a gift to you, not their job. Their time, energy, money, and food are all ways that they are showing love. Return that love in any way you can; a kind word, a note, a phone call. It can be hard when you don't feel well, but even the smallest gesture of thanks will mean a lot to someone who is trying to show they care! May God bless you through His laborers and may He bless all of them abundantly!

> *"Help should be helpful, not stressful!"*

"Above all, keep loving one another earnestly, since love covers a multitude of sins. Show hospitality to one another without grumbling. As each has received a gift, use it to serve one another, as good stewards of God's varied grace: whoever speaks, as one who speaks oracles of God; whoever serves, as one who serves by the strength that God supplies—in order that in everything God may be glorified through Jesus Christ." 1 Peter 4:8-10

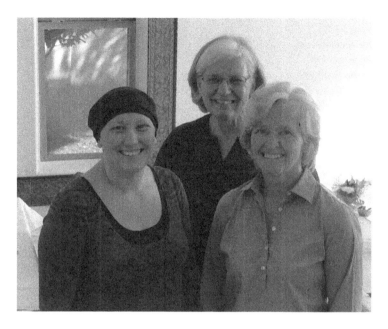

Laura with her mom, Ursula and
Aunt Corinne

But the fruit of the Spirit is love, joy, peace, patience, kindness, goodness,

faithfulness, gentleness, self-control; against such things there is no law "

Galatians 5:22-23

LAURA PENTSA

:CHAPTER 5:
MY NEW FRIEND, KING DAVID

B eing diagnosed with cancer, I was immediately hit with anxiety and fear. I quickly realized how little control I held in any aspect of life. I could not control if the medicine would work, I could not control whether the tumor would grow or shrink, and I could not control if I'd be here or well enough to plan my children's next birthday parties. I had NO control of those things. So what then? What could I do? What really mattered? These were the questions that really consumed my thoughts.

The simplest answer was: Praise the Lord! You may wonder how you praise while being plagued by fear? Is that even possible? Yes it is, and praise is powerful! It is healing to the mind and soul. You want proof? Take time to read a few Psalms and you will soon understand and learn from David. David who began as the little shepherd boy, then reigned as king, became an inspiring psalmist, and who was even described as a man after God's own heart. David lived an extreme life, but knew that he could run to the Lord in every circumstance. You too, can run to our Lord no matter what emotion you feel. You can pour out your heart openly, and honestly, expressing your every fear and need, and then Praise Him!

In His praise, I felt His love and His power, my fears were cast out, and my mountains were moved. In praise I also felt his presence and knew that I was not alone! When the Lord stands with you, all else seems small.

"I am the Alpha and the Omega," says the Lord God, "

who is and who was and who is to come, the Almighty" Revelation 1:8

Psalm 118 is one of my favorites because it gives a glimpse into eternity. ..."for His mercy endureth forever." FOREVER.... His mercy endureth FOREVER.... Just think about that for a second. His mercy is not just in this moment or just while you pray, but forever! Praise Him for that! Praise Him that you were created. Praise Him that He has blessed you with so much good here on Earth that you desire a cure and to live here even longer. Praise Him for all the gifts He has given you, like your friends and your family. Praise Him for your protection, your church, His Holy Word, His Only Son, His Spirit, and His plan of Salvation! There is so much more to Praise Him for. Take some time to think about all the ways he's begun to show you mercy. Now, just remember this is only the start, because His mercy endures FOREVER!

When you praise the Lord, for that time your mind and soul are set free of the burdens of this life and they are focused on Him, and that focus is the type of JOY that Apostle Paul writes about. Praising the Lord and finding peace in knowing that you are His and that He loves you is what really matters. No matter what today holds, cling to this truth that God is good. He is merciful. He is forever.

I would sometimes think about Heaven and what it will be like. The Bible gives some descriptions in the book of Revelation, but I would wonder about the differences and the similarities compared to Earth. Will anything be familiar? There are a couple things I am sure of: The Lord our God and Jesus Christ my Savior are the same today as they will be when I am there with them. I will still be praising them. They will still be my first love.

"Oh give thanks to the Lord, for he is good; for his steadfast love endures forever! Let Israel say, "His steadfast love endures forever." Let the house of Aaron say, "His steadfast love endures forever." Let those who fear the Lord say, "His steadfast love endures forever. "Out of my distress I called on the Lord; the Lord answered me and set me free. The Lord is on my side; I will not fear. What can man do to me? The Lord is on my side as my helper; I shall look in triumph on those who hate me. It is better to *take refuge in the Lord* than to trust in man. It is better to *take refuge in the Lord* than to trust in princes. All nations surrounded me; in the name of the Lord I cut them off! They surrounded me, surrounded me on every side; in the name of the Lord I cut them off! They surrounded me like bees; they went out like a fire among thorns; in the name of the Lord I cut them off! I was pushed hard, so that I was falling, but the Lord helped me. The Lord is my strength and my song; he has become my salvation. *Glad songs of salvation* are in the tents of the righteous: "The right hand of the Lord does valiantly, the right hand of the Lord exalts, the right hand of the *Lord does valiantly!*" I shall not die, but I shall live, and recount the deeds of the Lord. The Lord has disciplined me severely, but he has not given me over to death. Open to me the gates of righteousness, that I may enter through them and give thanks to the Lord. This is the gate of the Lord; the righteous shall enter through it. I thank you that you have answered me and have become my salvation. The stone that the builders rejected has become the cornerstone. This is the Lord's doing; it is marvelous in our eyes. This is the day that the Lord has made; let us rejoice and be glad in it. Save us, we pray, O Lord! O Lord, we pray, give us success! Blessed is he who comes in the name of the Lord! We bless you from the house of the Lord. The Lord is God, and he has made his light to shine upon us. Bind the festal sacrifice with cords, up to the horns of the altar! You are my God, and I will give thanks to you; you are my God; I will extol you. Oh give thanks to the Lord, for he is good; for his steadfast love endures forever!" Psalm 118

My first love. That is something that I had to really think about, too. I've always taught my kids that we are to love the Lord more than anyone or anything else. I've always tried to live this way, but I wondered, when I am in Heaven with the Lord, will my love and praise feel the same to Him? Will He know that He was always my first love? When I thought about this, my desire to praise Him and pour my heart out in song and prayer grew. My desire to intentionally show Him love actually deepened my love and faith in Him. Praise is one thing that you can begin today and know that you will still be doing throughout all of eternity.

"And from the throne came a voice saying, "Praise our God, all you his servants, you who fear him, small and great." Revelation 19:5

Though cancer may strip any semblance of control you once thought you had, there are still things you can do that matter. You can still praise, worship, and love Him. This will not only give God glory, but it will bring you a small glimpse of heaven here on Earth. This focus and desire puts all of the other struggles in perspective, for today is so very small when your sight is set on forever.

"...I have found in David the son of Jesse a man after my heart, who will do all my will." Acts 13:22b

How could David be a man after God's own heart? Could God also describe me that way? David did so much wrong. He sinned, he committed both adultery and murder, and yet this was the same man who God called a man after his own heart. Why did the Lord say this about David?

Well, David had a true love and trust in God, and though he did sin, he also repented. Psalm 51 is a beautiful view into David's heart. He knew that he was filthy and sinful, but had faith that the Lord's love and mercy could blot out every stain and renew him, purify him, and make him "whiter than snow". This is what sets David apart. His deep faith in God's steadfast love. This brings me so much comfort.

Having cancer, I sometimes felt guilty for having fear, having anxiety, being angry. Sometimes I wanted to do things my own way and in my own time, like David sometimes did. We are human, we are part of this Earthly, fallen world and we cannot be perfect. However, even with our imperfections, the Lord loves us and is merciful. Repenting of those things that are sinful or confessing my human struggles and thoughts to the Lord and then asking for His forgiveness and help renewed me. Follow David's example of repentance and praise:

"Have mercy on me, O God, according to your steadfast love; according to your abundant mercy blot out my transgressions. Wash me thoroughly from my iniquity, and cleanse me from my sin!" Psalm 51:1-2

Facing a battle with cancer, you will need courage. Where does your spirit's help come from? Where will you go to gather up courage? If you think wearing pink and putting on a smile is all it takes, it's only going to help for a fleeting moment. What gave me courage was knowing who is really fighting with me. I prayed and asked the Lord to fight this battle for me. I knew it was not something I could do, nor was I brave enough to even try it. The Lord gave me the strength to face every day and sometimes it was just one minute at-a-time.

One of my scariest times was going in for my first chemo infusion. I was scared of the process, I was scared of the side effects, I was scared that it wouldn't work.... yet, I was also excited... I was excited that it *could* work, and I was excited that my battle against the cancer was about to begin! I was ready, I was excited, but I was still scared!

I remembered the week prior to chemo, going through tons of tests, scans, and other physicals to be sure we knew what we were up against, and learning if my body was strong enough to go into battle. All through that week a song from my childhood kept coming to mind. It was a Sunday school song that I grew up singing but never anticipated how powerful and calming it would be when facing this sort of trial. The lyrics are:

Only a boy named David, only a little sling,
only a boy named David, **but he could pray and sing.**
Only a boy named David, only a rippling brook,
only a boy named David, but five little stones he took.
And one little stone went in the sling,
and the sling went round and round.
And one little stone went in the sling,
and the sling went round and round,
and round and round and round and round,
and round and round and round.
And one little stone went up in the air,
and **the giant came tumbling down.**

This song played over and over again in my head going into my first chemo. I remember thinking if this little shepherd boy David could walk up to the big nasty Goliath with only his faith and a sling shot, then how can I question anything going into my battle? I needed to trust that God would battle for me and that no matter what came of it, I only needed to trust Him. I felt like a warrior at my first chemo!

"Then David said to the Philistine, "You come to me with a sword and with a spear and with a javelin, but I come to you in the name of the Lord of hosts, the God of the armies of Israel, whom you have defied. This day the Lord will deliver you into my hand, and I will strike you down and cut off your head. And I will give the dead bodies of the host of the Philistines this day to the birds of the air and to the wild beasts of the earth, that all the earth may know that there is a God in Israel, and that all this assembly may know that the Lord saves not with sword and spear. For the battle is the Lord's, and he will give you into our hand." 1 Samuel 17:45-47

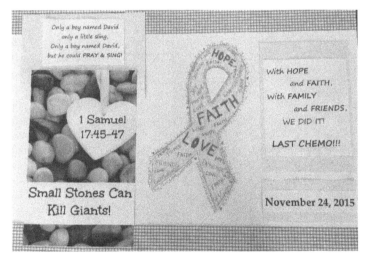

This was the poster I held up at the end of my last chemotherapy infusion!

:CHAPTER 6:
PRACTICAL ADVICE FOR CHEMOTHERAPY

The sound of a soft, soothing waterfall, coupled with big beautiful sunny windows that look out over a vast open desert and bright blue skies. Big comfy leather recliners, blankets, magazines, television, and hot coffee or tea at the ready. Doesn't sound like a bad way to pass a few hours, but nobody hopes to be on the waiting list to reserve these seats. My oncologist had a beautiful office and while I was thankful to go to such a nice facility, nobody really wants to be there.

Spending months side-by-side with other cancer patients taught me something that I never understood about cancer before; 'cancer' is a vague word. When someone has a stomach ache, people realize that there are many different reasons that could cause a stomach ache and many different ways to handle the problem. With a stomach ache, it could be caused by nerves, eating too much, eating the wrong thing, having the stomach flu, needing to use the restroom, acid, motion sickness, etc. Well, before I had cancer I naively thought that all cancers were somewhat similar, and that all treatments were somewhat similar. That is not true at all. The word cancer is vague, as it is a broad umbrella which encompasses so many forms, so many stages, and so many treatments.

I learned that even going to the same doctor and sitting side by side with someone getting chemotherapy at the same time as you, the similarities could very easily stop there. One of you may be feeling good that day and be ok to go about their day when the infusion is complete, while the other person may be home and in bed the remainder of the week. Some people have few side effects, while others seem to feel them all. I think

I was fortunate to fall somewhere in the middle. I would compare going through chemotherapy to a pregnancy; you can be in a room full of expectant mothers and each feels it differently, each has their own unique story to tell, and advice as to what worked to make them comfortable. I want to share with you my unique story and techniques that helped me get through chemotherapy. I am not a doctor or an expert, I only have knowledge based on my own personal experience. I sincerely hope some of this can help others, but I also know that each person must try different things to find what makes them most comfortable.

"He gives power to the faint, and to him who has no might he increases strength. Even youths shall faint and be weary, and young men shall fall exhausted; but they who wait for the Lord shall renew their strength; they shall mount up with wings like eagles; they shall run and not be weary; they shall walk and not faint." Isaiah 40:29-31

♡♡♡

The chemo regimen I was prescribed was quite aggressive; triple-negative breast cancer grows very fast and can spread quickly. I am very thankful mine did not spread! The entire tumor was confined to my right breast. I do think the chemotherapy my doctor prescribed helped to prevent any spreading. He prescribed a total of 16 infusions.

This was the breakdown of my chemotherapy infusions. For the first eight weeks, I would receive AC (doxorubicin & cyclophosphamide) every two weeks. After those four infusions were complete, I went to weekly doses of Taxol (Paclitaxel) with the addition of Carboplatin every three weeks.

So why is chemotherapy a good thing? In a nutshell, these drugs keep the cancer cells from dividing and growing. When effective, they can shrink and kill the cancer cells. In my case, I am thankful to say the drugs were very effective. I praise the Lord that He allowed this treatment to work for me!

♡♡♡

My Power Port

Before I began chemo, my doctors ordered a series of tests to ensure my body and heart could handle the medications. Another procedure prescribed was to have minor surgery to place a port. It makes blood draws and infusions so much easier. I recommend asking your doctor about your options.

A common misunderstanding is that when you have a port you won't feel the needle. This is not true, you still feel a stick, but it is fast and predictable. No trying this vein, and then that one. The bump under the skin is obvious to the nurses and usually one quick stick and it is done! They also have a numbing spray to use, and while it only numbs the very top layer of skin, I did think it was helpful. Recently someone told me that they asked for a tube of EMLA numbing cream and would cover their port area one hour before having it poked and they never felt a thing. While I never did this, I wish I had known. Ask your nurse if this is an option.

> *Tip: Try chewing gum or sucking on a mint while the port is flushed.*
> *It helps hide the bitter taste from saline.*

Only specific nurses are able to administer medications through a port, so you always need to make mention if you want your port used at a lab or hospital so that they can set you up with the right person. You will receive a card after the surgery with your port information and you must keep that with you. Mine actually came with a little card to hang on your keys, like a grocery reward program. I found that so strange and amusing, but it was actually genius, because once I did end up in the hospital unexpectedly and was glad to have it right there on my key chain.

One other tip is to chew gum or have a mint while your port is flushed with saline. My understanding is that not everyone can taste and smell the saline, but to me it was a very strong bitter taste. When I chewed gum I barely noticed it.

Getting a port put in was a bit scary for me. I had only been diagnosed that week so my mind was still processing everything. I had only been in for surgery one other time - a cesarean section delivery with my youngest daughter, which is a very different story. So, when I got there I was a bundle of nerves. My very kind nurse Jim could see how tense I was, and he helped me relax by telling me exactly what to expect. He told me some positive stories of other cancer survivors he knew and that when this whole treatment was over, he hoped he'd be the nurse on staff when my port came out. He wanted to dance in celebration and victory that day when it was all behind me. He was such a blessing to me that day! Many times in the months to follow I'd visualize finishing treatment and dancing with him in celebration. He gave me something to really hope for. I tear up just thinking of what a gift he was to me!

The actual procedure proved anti-climactic. I should not have been scared. Basically, they got me all set up in a gown with an IV, just like any other test or procedure, but when they took me into the surgery room they administered a twilight medicine which makes everything just fade away. I could still see and hear, but I just didn't care! I remember seeing a blinking number on the monitor in front of me and thinking it was funny because I didn't know what a number was anymore. I just kept staring at it. My brain knew it was a number, but what did that even mean? I remember voices, but I couldn't understand them and I could feel my body being moved, but I couldn't feel any pain or tell what was happening. I have no idea if this was a normal "twilight reaction" but that is all I recall. There was no pain, no fear, and no difficulty.

When the procedure was done, I went back to the post-surgery area and rested a little bit. Nurse Jim brought me some food and reminded me that it is so important to eat. So I did and he smiled. He gave me some very important information that day: when getting ready to begin chemotherapy, he said "just eat!" He had seen many patients lose their appetite or only want to eat the perfect healthy choice, but didn't like it so they would get too thin and not have the strength to battle. He told me to "Just eat!", "Eat what you want, when you want it! If it is healthy even better!" "Just eat!". Later on, that tip made a lot of sense and it really was some of the best advice I ever received.

> **Tip: Just Eat!**

So my port was in. I couldn't go swimming for a while, and had to cover it in the shower for a couple days, but aside from that I can assure you it was well worth the procedure. I recommend talking to your oncologist about the pros and cons of ports for your particular treatment plan and condition. I no longer have my port, and I strangely miss it. Every time I need a blood draw I wish my port was still there. I never would have thought that a port would be something I'd miss.

Below are my Facebook posts from the week after diagnosis.

June 29th (Dave's birthday & 1st day at the new hospital!) Thank you to all who prayed and have been encouraging me. After a long morning of appointments, we have a plan of attack. At this point we think it is only the one mass & it is early enough that treatment should be effective. The plan begins with having a port placed next week and start chemotherapy the week following. Please continue praying & I will update as specific requests come up.

Love to you all! –Laura

June 30th It is the first step of treatment tomorrow. I am very thankful they can get started so quickly. I will be getting the port placed at 10am. Please pray that it goes smoothly & that it will heal well without any infection. Thank you all!!!

July 1st Port is in! I feel good! God blessed me with an amazing godly nurse who was such a blessing to me today! Feeling thankful! Thank you nurse Jim!

July 13th Today is my pet scan, praying that it confirms that there is only one lump and the cancer has not spread. After this, I should be allowed to start chemo. Hoping to start tomorrow or Wednesday. Ready to do this! Romans 15:13 May the God of hope fill you with all joy and peace in believing, so that by the power of the Holy Spirit you may abound in hope.

♡♡♡

Chemotherapy

Every dose of chemotherapy proved to result in a different experience with different side effects depending on which drugs were administered. However, the chemotherapy day routine was usually quite predictable. I was able to have chemotherapy infusions right inside my oncology office. It is a small staff so I quickly knew most of them. I loved feeling like I belonged there and that I didn't feel like a stranger. I felt comforted by their familiar faces.

A typical infusion began by choosing my chair amongst the row of other patients. I would get myself and a friend set up with our drinks and reading materials. My nurse would come and ask about my week, how I was tolerating treatment, update any medical data, and review my blood work results from the previous day. The doctor would sometimes stop by and check in with me, too.

My nurse would administer all necessary drugs via my port. I sometimes received Benadryl with my chemotherapy, and on those days I would get quite sleepy and doze off for a bit. Most of the time I would simply spend quiet, quality time conversing with my friend.

The infusion did not hurt. I could sometimes feel the cold medicine flowing through my veins, but a warm blanket helped. Otherwise, it was usually very calm and quiet. Chemotherapy day was not frightening or hard. In fact, I always made sure to take a picture during chemotherapy before any of the side effects began and I still felt well. The process usually took between 2-4 hours.

Immediately after leaving I would eat a hearty lunch, because I knew that everything would taste badly and the nausea would set in by evening. I would usually pick whatever restaurant or food I was in the mood for, and I would really savor and enjoy it. The day of infusion was usually not a bad day at all.

By that evening, going into the next couple days though, I usually felt pretty terrible. Those days were almost always spent in bed. Then I would make slow steady progress over the next few days until I felt reasonably well.

Talking to other patients I was shocked by how extreme their experiences could be. I remember talking to a few people who worked full time throughout their entire treatment and really didn't feel very many side effects at all. While I was thankful to be a stay-at-home mom and not have to worry about going into work, I honestly know that I could not have managed anything close. Then on the other extreme, I saw people who had been hospitalized, sometimes requiring a wheelchair and needing blood transfusions to keep going. I was sad that they suffered, and seeing their struggles helped me not to complain too much.

The further into treatment I went, the weaker my body was. I could feel my muscles losing strength and my energy level decreasing. It was the most physically trying time of my life and at times it did feel nearly impossible. Sometimes, it felt incomprehensible that drugs which cause so much damage were actually life saving. It seemed unlikely that I'd ever feel completely well again. It was hard to imagine ever finishing treatment.

While it was all hard to believe, it really was still something that I did believe. I did trust that all of those good things could happen! When I kept a positive perspective, treatment went much better.

I felt so much excitement and elation on my final, 16th infusion. I had done it! Even though I had never desired to take this path, reaching this monumental point felt like such a huge accomplishment! Following, you will see me pictured, holding up my poster in celebration of my last day of chemotherapy. I felt like an Olympic winner holding up my medal! It was a wonderful victorious day. Thank you Lord, for giving me the courage and strength to face each day!

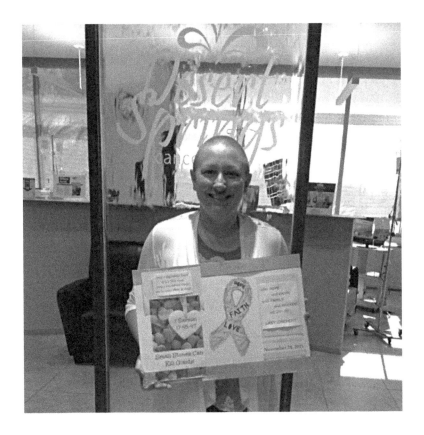

♡♡♡

Side Effects of Chemotherapy and How I Dealt with Them

Taste:

This was the change that remained nearly the whole course of treatment. Everything just tasted weird! Sometimes it was worse than others, but in general everything tasted like it came from a tin can with a metallic aftertaste. The day or two following my first AC treatment, things sometimes tasted pickled. It was strange. Certain things taste OK pickled like with a hamburger, you kind of expect pickles on it so it's not too bad, but when you are eating grilled chicken or maybe an apple and it tastes pickled, let's just say, it is really hard to get down. With nurse Jim's, "just eat" advice ringing in my ears. I didn't really let my taste buds stop me. Fortunately, that pickle thing lasted only a few days. The metallic tastes were more common for me and eventually I kind of got used to it.

The hardest thing for me was to drink water. It did not taste good and actually nauseated me. Did you know that when going through chemo you need to drink even more water? It is very easy to dehydrate, so it is important to find ways to make water appealing! Here are some ways to get fluid in, when water is not appealing.

-Propel mix. I loved these little dry pouches of Propel mix. I'd use one packet in a huge 32oz water bottle. The flavor was mild, but it took away that metallic taste. Plus, chemotherapy can sometimes lower the amount of electrolytes in the body so using Propel helped replenish them. Gatorade or other sports drinks can do the same thing, but I liked that I could add this dry mix to make the concentration to my liking. Later into treatment, my nurse even commented that my electrolytes were keeping up especially well on my blood tests and I believe this drink had helped.

-Lemons. there are some great health benefits to adding lemon to your water! Adding lemon to your water is a great way of getting your body more alkaline. Some say that keeping your body at a healthy alkaline chemistry can ward off cancer. I'm not an expert in the field, but there are many books on the topic. Also, lemons are a natural way to flush toxins out. Plus, they just taste great. Again, it's another favorite way to help hide the metallic taste.

-Green tea. I did not drink this daily, but when I was in the mood for something different, green tea with a bit of honey either hot or iced was comforting.

> *Tip: Keep a journal of your side effects. It will help you predict patterns and help your doctor to see what you are experiencing.*

Nausea:

This was a big problem for me on AC, but not as much on the carboplatin or taxol. I was given three days worth of anti-nausea meds during my infusions and still needed to take anti-nausea pills every few hours for the first two days after an AC infusion. Unfortunately the anti-nausea pills came with their own set of side effects for me, so I tried to stop them as soon as I could. Staying ahead of the nausea was critical. Once it got too bad (vomiting), it was hard to get it under control. Most of the time I never got to the stage of vomiting, because my anti-nausea drugs kept it from getting to that point. Even so, the nausea was often still there, feeling sick to my stomach and just extremely uncomfortable for a couple of days after AC infusions.

Another aide for nausea are the acupressure wrist bands. Waterproof adjustable bands that you wear like a watch. They have a hard dome that puts light pressure on the pressure point which helped ease nausea. A nurse friend of mine gave me a set as a gift and I really liked them.

Strangely, I found a really amazing anti-nausea technique that worked for me: my box of greeting cards! Seriously, it actually really helped! When I would be feeling very nauseous I would get out my box of cards. People would send cards with well wishes and scripture and I was amazed at how pulling out that box and really looking at each card

> *Reading the scripture on greeting cards was comforting, like being spoon-fed scripture one verse at a time.*

brought a cheerful distraction. Sometimes I'd just look at the picture and think about why they picked that picture for the card, or sometimes I'd reread all the handwritten notes inside the cards, or most often I'd look for the scripture verses and think about why those verses were chosen for comfort or encouragement.

The scripture verses were short, and it was like comforting spoonfuls of nourishment to my soul. It usually was the perfect distraction for those really uncomfortable times. I looked at them until I fell asleep or the discomfort subsided. I don't think I will ever be able to get rid of that box of cards. I still keep it in my closet where I see it every day.

Dry Mouth:

I found a brand called Biotene that had some wonderful products to help with dry mouth. They make a spray and mouthwash that really helped. In the same section of the drugstore you can find little melt away tablets that are fantastic. The little tablets were perfect to take in my purse or keep on my night stand. I only had a couple mouth sores, but rinsing with the mouthwash often really seemed to help the best. I was given a recipe for a helpful rinse: Mix the following ingredients in a 1 quart jar: 1 tsp of baking soda with 1 tsp of salt. Rinsing with this a couple times a day can keep your mouth clean and lower the risk of infection.

Dry Skin:

Chemo skin becomes very sensitive and dry. I found that coconut oil was a great way to moisturize my skin multiple times per day. I also found several natural balms and body butters that were rich and helpful to my poor dry skin. Strangely my face has never been clearer or more blemish-free than during chemotherapy. My face hardly needed any hydrating cream so I only used a bit of coconut oil. My feet were the complete opposite, often cracking and remaining difficult to keep hydrated. Overall, I would recommend staying with a good quality natural cream. Ingredients I like to read on the label are aloe, coconut and shea. I also preferred something very mild scented because strong lotions sometimes made the nausea worse.

Lip Balm was in high demand during that time and I found that I really liked lip balm with vitamin E or Shea. My personal favorite are the EOS brand, egg-shaped lip balms. They are smooth and made with Shea and Jojoba oil.

Pale Skin:

It seems that most chemo patients seem to get a bit washed out during treatment. I couldn't believe what a touch of bronzer could do. People were always telling me that I looked "so healthy" and had a "glow". Well, I know it was probably the bronzer, but I'd much rather hear those things, even if untrue, than have people look at me with sad eyes. A little bronzer, eye brow makeup, and lip gloss can do amazing things!

Nail changes:

I heard terrifying stories of women losing their nails during chemotherapy and am relieved that I did not lose any of mine. They did go through some changes, though. They were very dry and brittle so I always kept them trimmed quite short so that they wouldn't break or tear. My toe nails did get yellow and it was interesting to see the discoloration grow out when treatment was over. I developed a couple brown lines in my finger nails and one never went away. It still grows with one brown stripe that reminds me of all that I've been through. I avoided painting my nails during that time, not because of the polish, but because of the acetone to remove it. A nurse once told me that the acetone is really hard on chemo patients and she thought that might contribute to some people losing their nails. I don't know if that is fact, but I thought I'd rather have natural nails for a while than no nails, so I erred on the side of caution. I also used Vitamin E cuticle oil from time to time to help keep hydrated.

Neuropathy:

Neuropathy can happen when chemotherapy causes nerve damage. The extent of damage can vary tremendously from one person to another, but often is felt first in the outermost extremities like fingers and toes. I think Taxol was the chemo that brought about neuropathy for me because I really didn't notice any numbness or tingling until about the last month of chemo. My nutritional counselor had recommended taking Alpah Lipoic Acid and B-Complex vitamins to reduce and minimize neuropathy and I think they did help, because my symptoms were very mild and disappeared as soon as chemo ended. Sometimes when I am cold the neuropathy will resurface, but it usually doesn't last long.

Fatigue:

Chemo and the side effects left me very weak and tired at times. I found long naps could make sleeping at night really difficult which only worsened the fatigue, but small cat naps could often help get me through the day. Even just laying down to rest without sleeping could sometimes get me by. I tried to keep my body fueled with small healthy meals and snacks throughout the day. If I really didn't want to eat, I'd gulp down a nutritional supplement like Ensure. I didn't love the taste, but I knew that I needed to provide my body fuel and energy. I'd take time for short naps, and sometimes that meant asking for help with the household tasks like cooking and cleaning. I learned to save my energy for the things I had to do, or for the things I loved to do. Sometimes living out of a clean laundry basket was ok too, if it meant having the energy to interact with the family. I had to pick and choose where my energy would be used.

Hormone Changes:

Wow, hot flashes! I always thought that was just an exaggeration, a perfect running joke, a short phase that women hit during menopause. To all of you suffering from hot flashes, I am so so sorry. It is real, it is frustrating, and it is out and out annoying! A few ways I learned to deal with these were to wear breathable fabrics, keep a fan near the bed, keep wipes on the night stand to give a quick, instant cooling effect, and if the wipes didn't work, I'd get up and step into a cold bath. That was my last resort, because it's difficult to go back to sleep after that. My sister-in-law also bought me an instant cool towel; I'd wet it in cold water and it slowly evaporated keeping me cool. I used this a lot in my car, and it helped keep me cool without freezing my kids with the air conditioner. Hormone changes can also cause early menopause or just temporarily stop your cycle. I am one year post chemo now, and things are still not back to normal. Be patient and cut yourself a break because hormone changes are a big deal and they affect your body in many ways. If you are concerned about your hormonal changes, call your doctor.

Feeling Cold:

On the opposite side of hot flashes, there were times when my body felt so cold, usually during or right after an infusion. A pair of cozy socks and a soft blanket were perfect for this. Actually my fantastic niece Aubrey, made me a soft felt blanket to take to every infusion for this very reason. The medicine they put through the IV can feel cold and having a blanket is a really good idea.

Constipation:

Embarrassing to discuss. However, constipation was my worst side effect. There were a couple of instances that I worried this problem might even land me in the ER. I was never sure if this side effect was directly because of chemo or if it was due to anti-nausea medicine or antihistamine drugs. But whatever the reason, the problem was real! I found that it took some real trial and error to get things just right. I won't go into great detail, (you're welcome), but I will list some things you might want to keep in the cupboard.

Stool softeners, fiber supplements, and gentle laxatives (pills) are good choices for mild issues or to just keep everything moving. Smooth lax (powder) is an option for bigger problems. Then there's magnesium citrate (liquid) for really concerning problems! I would also recommend getting witch hazel pads to help keep everything clean and soothed. Hemorrhoid suppositories may be needed, and Dermoplast pain relieving spray proved to be very valuable.

> *This recipe is full of fiber and helped when I was having trouble.*
> ***Prune Applesauce:***
> *1/3 cup applesauce*
> *1/3 cup baby prunes or prune juice*
> *1/3 cup bran*
> *Mix together or blend. Store in the refrigerator and eat 1-2 tbls in the evening with a 4-8 oz glass of water.*

Red Fluids:

It is gross and at first a bit alarming, but completely normal for AC chemotherapy (AC is sometimes nicknamed the "red devil") which can turn your urine, sweat or even tears red immediately following infusion. It is not dangerous, it just looks really strange. Thankfully my chemo nurse Jen warned me this would happen, otherwise I may have fainted in the restroom! When I was getting AC infusions I tried to just drink a lot of water that day and usually the color was all flushed out by bedtime.

Risk of Infection:

Toward the end of my chemotherapy, my white blood cell counts were dangerously low. I was warned that without Neupogen shots to boost my cell count I might end up needing a transfusion or end up in the hospital. With low white blood cell counts comes a much higher risk of infection. I took advice to stay away from public areas when possible for the last few weeks of chemotherapy and try to stay healthy. Was it fun to stay home and not attend social gatherings? NO. Was it a good idea? Yes! While it was not a guarantee that I would not catch something, I wanted to do all I could to keep from ending up in the hospital. I had made it through almost all of the infusions and I did not want to delay the end of treatment. Sometimes you have to look at the big picture and make hard decisions that are what is best for you.

> *I realize for some of you staying away from the public is not an option, but if you can help it, when your white blood counts are in trouble avoid extra trips to the store, going into busy crowded places. Stay home when you can, fill your body with good nutritious food, rest and let yourself heal!*

While you may not have these same side effects, I hope that *if* you do, I've given you some tools to help find comfort and ease your way through the discomfort.

Below are some of the gifts that I loved and would give to anyone else about to go into chemotherapy.

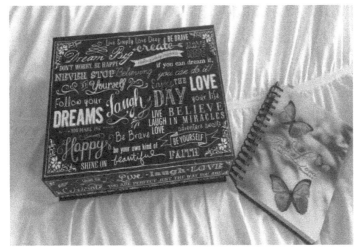

Above: My mom went shopping with me the week I was diagnosed and she got me a box to hold all of the cards of encouragement that I received with a journal to write down all the "good" stuff that comes from this situation. Things I actually want to remember. I have pages of scribbled down little blessings and "God sightings". Reading back through the journal and cards on hard days brings about peace and strength.

Right: I called this gift my "dollar store box of sanity". It was a bin filled with lots of inexpensive crafts that the kids can do with me in bed. Easy 5 minute crafts that take no prep and minimal clean up. This was a great gift! I was feeling a lot of guilt when I couldn't go do stuff with the 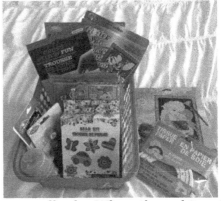 kids, or couldn't play like we normally do. When those bits of guilt popped up, we'd grab the sanity bin and do a little craft on the couch or even in bed. Once people saw how much we used these type of gifts, people just kept replenishing the box.

Below: My friends threw me a mini pre-chemo party, the day before chemo started and gave me a tote bag signed with encouragement. It says fight like a girl on the other side. I carried it to chemotherapy each treatment. They each brought chemo care gifts. Lip gloss, lotion, Biotene Dry mouth, nose & eye care, nausea drops, scarves, reading material, blankets etc... It was so thoughtful and practical.

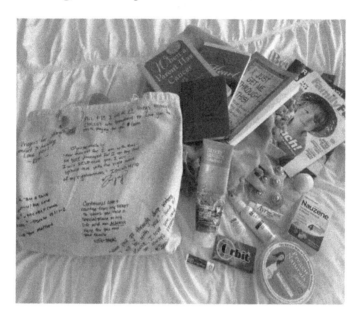

"... give, and it will be given to you. Good measure, pressed down, shaken together, running over, will be put into your lap. For with the measure you use it will be measured back to you." Luke 6:38

More gifts I would recommend for chemo patients or anyone with limited mobility.

❖ I loved receiving the magazine subscription to "life:beautiful". It arrives seasonally and has beautiful photography and incredibly inspiring articles. Beautiful, colorful magazines are a great gift idea.

❖ Music CD's or ITunes gift cards. Worship music was a treasure!

❖ Happy, uplifting movies and tv-shows. A list of your personal favorites and recommendations with the reason why you liked them is wonderful.

❖ I hesitate to say it, but money. Cancer is so expensive! We received cards in the mail with cash gifts and we were incredibly appreciative.

❖ Groceries. Meals were great too, but groceries were so nice to have on hand and ready for the family.

❖ A housekeeper. Having someone clean is fantastic, but I felt awkward when friends cleaned for me. A stranger was completely different though. I was able to find a local cleaning service that helps women during chemotherapy for FREE with a once a month cleaning. It was amazing! Look into this for your friend and see if there is one in their area. If not, perhaps you can afford to pay for a professional cleaner to come in once or weekly.

❖ Flowers. I love flowers and they really did cheer me up.

❖ Lots of cards. Texts are great, but a card is lasting. It shows effort and thought. It can be left out to look at or kept for another day.

:CHAPTER 7:
CHEMOTHERAPY - IN FAST FORWARD

A s a way to document my journey, I took a picture at all 16 of my chemotherapy infusions. I purposefully asked different friends to accompany me to my infusions, not because they are difficult or scary, but because it made me look forward to the day. I was able to have quiet, quality time with these friends while I did something that other-wise would have been a chore. It strengthened our bonds and helped them to

> **Tip: Find ways to include friends during this time. It will be a blessing to you both.**

understand what I was going through. Having these friends join me made each infusion different and memorable. I think it was one of my best decisions while I had cancer.

The following pages are full of smiling pictures I took each morning of chemotherapy. It was easy to smile because I usually felt at my peak, at my very best of the week just before the infusion. All of the side effects from the last infusion were starting to fade. It was easy to smile because I was so hopeful that the medicine would do its job and that with God's help I would be healed. It was easy to smile because my friends were with me. I was in good company!

I often struggled with the fact that I didn't take pictures during the days that followed. The days when I was too sleepy to get out of my pajamas, or too nauseous to take a shower. I struggled feeling hypocritical, taking pictures only on the easy smiling day, and not on the rough hard days. I chose to do this though, because it was so difficult at that time to be so completely public while I was still sick. I didn't want people focused on my hard days. I wanted them to know I was having good days. I didn't want my sick picture to circulate and cause worry or panic when I knew that I would bounce back.

I didn't want people to say anything sad or scary to my kids who were already living it. So for those reasons (and more), I mostly posted pictures of my good days. I tried to be very honest with my posts and express my overall emotions and prayer requests, but the pictures to me were different. So, please observe a very speedy, fast forward look through my five months of chemotherapy!

"You keep him in perfect peace whose mind is stayed on you,

because he trusts in you Trust in the Lord forever,

for the Lord God is an everlasting rock."

Isaiah 26:3-4

FIRST CHEMO: July 14th"Only a boy named David, only a little sling, only a boy named David, but he could PRAY & SING" The last couple weeks this song has stayed with me. When I think of the battle ahead, I am comforted to know that this battle belongs to the Lord! May God allow these first chemo drugs to be as effective as David's little stone! I appreciate every prayer, they are encouraging me and strengthening me!

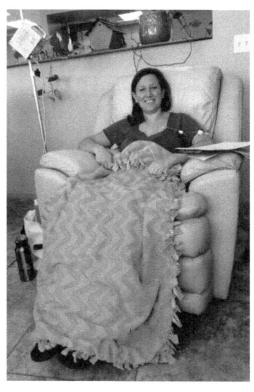

"The prayer of a righteous man is powerful and effective." James 5:16

July 14th (on drive home after 1st chemo)

1st chemo is done! Feeling good and I am glad the plan is IN ACTION! Now, just taking it day by day.

July 17:

Well, I think I am finally on the up side of chemo round one. It was a very yucky couple of days, but not as bad as I'd expected. I am very grateful for anti-nausea medicine and dry mouth remedies, however so much more I am so thankful for our moms! One mom busy cooking and cleaning, the other making sure I stay on top of my medicine and ready to help with whatever I need. Both teaming up to make sure the kids are loved and cared for and that our house still feels like home. Thank you both for your love and taking such good care of my precious family! If I hadn't felt so yucky, I may have actually felt spoiled!

"Love is patient and kind; love does not envy or boast; it is not arrogant or rude. It does not insist on its own way; it is not irritable or resentful; it does not rejoice at wrongdoing, but rejoices with the truth. Love bears all things, believes all things, hopes all things, endures all things." 1 Corinthians 13:4-7

July 28th

Round 2!!! Here with great company, my cousin and life long friend!

"The LORD will fight for you; you need only to be still"

Exodus 14:14

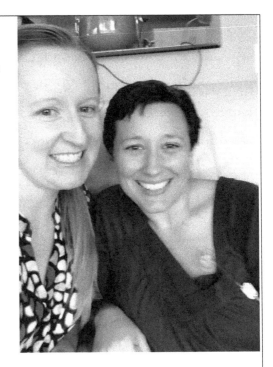

August 6th

Bless The Lord, Oh My Soul!

What a beautiful day!!! I am celebrating and full of praise!! Eight years ago, God answered my cries for a child, my sweet boy was born. I love that kid, he makes me laugh and brings me so much joy! Then God blessed me beyond what I'd asked and gave me my two sweet girls without any waiting. I am thankful for my family! In addition, I am full of praise today for another answered prayer: my oncologist confirmed what I was already suspecting, the CANCER IS significantly SHRINKING!!! God has allowed this chemo to be extremely effective, and I am overwhelmed with thanks!

Cancer and chemo prove to be hard and bring new challenges daily, but knowing that it is working makes it so so worth it!!! So many verses run through my mind today it is hard to pick just one, so I'll share just these two with you. If you'd like to share a verse with me, I'd love to read them, just note it in the comments.

Ephesians 3:12 In Christ we can come before God with freedom and without fear. We can do this through faith in Christ

Matthew 7:7-8 "Ask, and it will be given to you; seek, and you will find; knock, and it will be opened to you. For everyone who asks receives, and the one who seeks finds, and to the one who knocks it will be opened."

Aug 11th: Chemo #3: Knowing that the medicine is working makes coming in much easier. Plus, I have Jenn here! One of 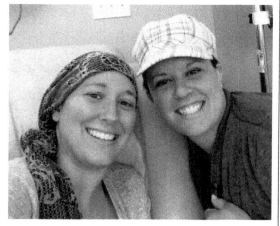 the best perks of marriage was adding sisters to my life! I love this girl!

"For the mountains may depart and the hills be removed, but my steadfast love shall not depart from you, and my covenant of peace shall not be removed" says the Lord, who has compassion on you." Isaiah 54:10

Aug 25th

Look who is here with me today! My Adrienne! I am so blessed to have her and so many others supporting me, loving me and praying for me! Thank you all for lifting me up! Chemo #4 is underway and it is the final dose of AC chemo! In two weeks I begin my 12 consecutive

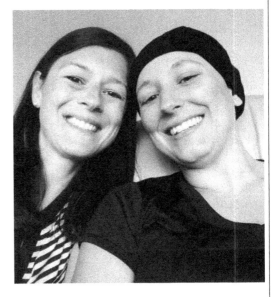

weeks of taxol and carboplatin chemo. Again, heading into the unknown and praying God will give me the strength needed each day, and that He will allow me complete healing.

"Two are better than one, because they have a good reward for their toil. For if they fall, one will lift up his fellow. But woe to him who is alone when he falls and has not another to lift him up!"
Ecclesiastes 4:9-10

Sept 8th: Chemo #5! Starting new medicines today, mixed emotions about that, but overall very thankful that God is taking me step by step.
Annette is here with me, supporting me just as she has always done. As long as I can remember I've always known she loves me like family; what a true friend! Romans 12:12

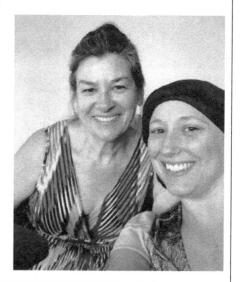

"Rejoice in hope, be patient in tribulation, be constant in prayer."

Sept 15th: Chemo #6! My brother Steve is here cheering me on and making me laugh! Love him even more and more all the time! I wanted to share a song that I love with all of you today. I first heard this song about a month ago, and it has become a special part of my day. In times that I feel weak, this song is the perfect prayer of worship from me to my Great God. When I sing it, I can feel Him so close, and I know He is with me. I hope it brings all

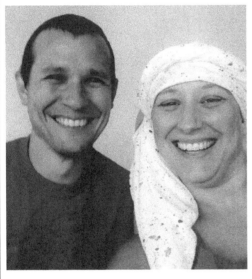

of you peace and joy! (song lyrics on pg. 127)

"For I am sure that neither death nor life, nor angels nor rulers, nor things present nor things to come, nor powers, nor height nor depth, nor anything else in all creation, will be able to separate us from the love of God in Christ Jesus our Lord." Romans 8:38-39

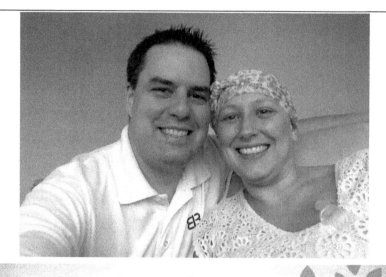

As a **Husband** I will:
love, lead, and provide
- Ephesians 5:25-29
- I Corinthians 11:3
- I Timothy 5:8

As a **Wife** I will:
help, manage, and love
- Genesis 2:18, 21-22
- I Timothy 5:14
- Titus 2:4

"Two are better than one" Eccl. 4:9

September 22nd

Chemo #7! Dave is with me,

always a blessing to me!

I love this picture and am so thankful that he was by my side every day, not just one chemotherapy! Dave, I love you!

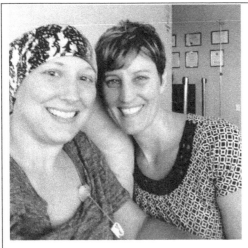

Sept 29th: Chemo #8 of 16, YES, that means I'm halfway through chemo!!! Here with Jackie today, she has been with me this week and I love having her here. She is the big cousin I always looked up to as a kid and I still think she is pretty cool. So thankful she could come and be with me! Yesterday, worry started to creep in and this verse soothed my soul. God's word is healing. Praise the Lord oh my soul.

"Blessed is the man who trusts in the Lord, whose trust is the Lord. He is like a tree planted by water, that sends out its roots by the stream, and does not fear when heat comes, for its leaves remain green, and is not anxious in the year of drought, for it does not cease to bear fruit." Jeremiah 17:7-8

Oct 6th

Chemo #9. Here today with Karen! From hand sewn satin pillow cases and port cushions to a really thoughtful tote bag signed by our friends, she has been showing me love and encouragement!

2 Corinthians 12:9

"But he said to me, "My grace is sufficient for you, for my power is made perfect in weakness." Therefore I will boast all the more gladly of my weaknesses, so that the power of Christ may rest upon me."

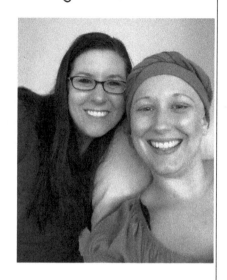

Oct 6th:

I thought I'd send out some health updates as I had a very informative Dr. appointment today after chemo. First of all, very full of praise that this chemo has been so very effective. During a quick exam the Dr. couldn't find the tumor at all today which means by the time surgery comes we have a very good hope of every last cancer cell being eradicated. If that hope is found true during the mastectomy pathology report, then he said there is a very good chance that radiation will NOT be necessary. This would cut my treatment back by months!!! So thankful for the chemo working!.... Now, that said, chemo attacks all fast growing cells, the bad and unfortunately also the good. My white and red blood counts have been quite low the last 2-3 weeks. Last week I had to go in daily for shots to bring the white counts up. It worked, but I am still very "borderline". I've been advised to keep public outings to a minimum and do my best to keep healthy. A cold or flu could land me in the hospital very fast. Also, I'm learning that the carboplatin chemo is very, very hard on me, so next time I get that I'll be asking for more specific prayer requests. So... my dear friends you may not see me around for a bit, I will be "hiding" at home and loving on my precious family. Visitors will be at a minimum for a while, and if you have any sign of illness please lets take a rain check. This is just part of chemo, but I am over half way through, 9 down 7 more to go!

Thank you for all your prayers, I am blessed and loved beyond measure.

Philippians 4:6-7 Do not be anxious about anything, but in everything by prayer and supplication with thanksgiving let your requests be made known to God. And the peace of God, which surpasses all understanding, will guard your hearts and your minds in Christ Jesus.

Oct 13th : Chemo #10! I've had the privilege of watching this sweet little girl grow into an amazing and talented woman! So happy Melaney could be with me today! Verse 11 helped me through our move to AZ and is just as calming during this trial. Verses 12-13 are verses I think everyone can cling to on the best or worst of days. Beautiful living word! Jeremiah 29:11-13

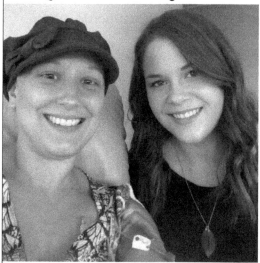

"11 For I know the plans I have for you, declares the Lord, plans for welfare and not for evil, to give you a future and a hope. 12 Then you will call upon me and come and pray to me, and I will hear you. 13 You will seek me and find me, when you seek me with all your heart."

Chemo #11: Here with Mom. Vickie flew out for the second time since I was diagnosed to help the family.

She shows love through her devotion to us, and her desire to serve. I'm thankful she is here, and thankful that Dad shares her with us!

I'll need prayer support this week as I'm getting carboplatin with my taxol today, plus daily white-blood count shots. I've gotta say I really hope carbo does it's job, because I am not fond of it! I've had it twice and both times experienced something that cannot be summed up into a tidy two word side effect 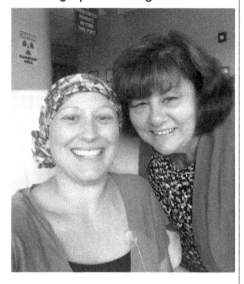 warning label. Bare with me as I attempt to describe... Both times I've had this, I am SO WEAK, and SO EXHAUSTED that things get a little nutty. My soul, body and mind start competing for the leading role and it feels scary. My body starts complaining and pointing out every annoyance, my mind starts to wander and "go down the rabbit hole", while my soul tries to coax the other two back into submission. I feel disconnected and conflicted for a couple days. It feels scary. Please pray that my soul can take the lead and that I can sleep through those times when my body is so bone tired that it only wants to cause trouble. I don't want to complain, but I honestly need the prayer support, so I am willing to be vulnerable and open up about this. Thanks everyone!

"In you, O Lord, do I take refuge; let me never be put to shame!

In your righteousness deliver me and rescue me; incline your ear to me, and save me! Be to me a rock of refuge, to which I may continually come; you have given the command to save me, for you are my rock and my fortress" Psalm 71: 1-3

Oct 23rd

Lots to be thankful for today! Dave & I celebrate our 16th wedding anniversary!!!! I am feeling better after this week's chemo and on the upside. And... hundreds of itty bitty things to be thankful for...

MY HAIR... it is starting to grow back!
From the biggest to the smallest, we are blessed!

Oct 27th Chemo #12 (Getting Taxol, my personal favorite). Only 4 more chemos to go after today! My very true and loyal friend Stephanie is with me, like she is so often. She drives me for blood work and helps with the kids' homework every week. She's always coming up with ways to

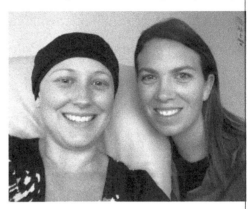

help and creative solutions. I am so thankful for her! "Come to me, all you who are weary and burdened, and I will give you rest. Take my yoke upon you and learn from me, for I am gentle and humble in heart, and you will find rest for your souls. For my yoke is easy and my burden is light."
Matthew 11:28-30

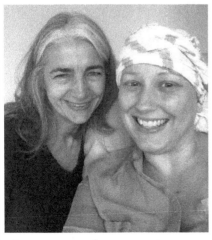

Nov 3rd: Chemo #13. My Aunt Marta is here supporting me. She always gives 110% to everything she cares about, she is enthusiastic and diligent. I consider myself very blessed that she cares about me!

"Whatever you do, work heartily, as for the Lord and not for men, knowing that from the Lord you will receive the inheritance as your reward. You are serving the Lord Christ." Colossians 3:23-24

Chemo #14! Enjoying today with my cousin Denise by my side. She is an amazing friend, someone who is so much fun to be silly with, but also knows just what to say when things get serious. Incredibly encouraging and a constant prayer warrior, I'm so glad she is in my life! Today is my last "yucky" chemo! Hoping this will be the last time I EVER need 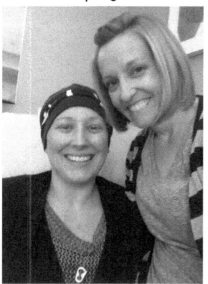 to take Carboplatin. Then just two Taxol's to go!!! That said, I must thank all of you for your prayers during the last Carboplatin. I was comforted knowing I was cared for and was able to rest much better. Just before my diagnosis, I was studying the book of Esther and was deeply impacted by the fact that Esther went to her people and asked them to fast on her behalf so she could courageously go before the king. That passage helped me to ask for all of your help, and I cannot thank you enough for being my people. God continues to strengthen me to be strong and courageous. If any of you have specific prayer requests today or ever, call or message me, I want to be your people too!

"Then Esther told them to reply to Mordecai, "Go, gather all the Jews to be found in Susa, and hold a fast on my behalf, and do not eat or drink for three days, night or day. I and my young women will also fast as you do. Then I will go to the king, though it is against the law, and if I perish, I perish." Mordecai then went away and did everything as Esther had ordered him." Esther 4: 15-17 (For any of my friends who don't know this book, don't worry, she does not perish, and God does save her people! It's a great book!)

Nov 17: Chemo # 15!!! Almost done! I've been looking forward to today, just so I can have some quality time with Michelle. We never have enough time together and I so enjoy her sincerity peppered with the most surprising sense of humor. Today will

be fun. I can't believe how much support I've had,
and how much it
has helped turn a
difficult 15 weeks
into something
beautiful. So many
people showing
they care, not only
with me at chemo,
but helping with

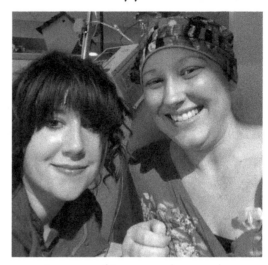

the kids, bringing groceries, sending cards, and so
many other ways. I am blessed with amazing friends
and family! "This is the message we have heard
from him and proclaim to you, that God is light,
and in him is no darkness at all. If we say we have
fellowship with him while we walk in darkness, we
lie and do not practice the truth. But if we walk in
the light, as he is in the light, we have fellowship
with one another, and the blood of Jesus his Son
cleanses us from all sin. If we say we have no sin, we
deceive ourselves, and the truth is not in us. If we
confess our sins, he is faithful and just to forgive us
our sins and to cleanse us from all unrighteousness.
If we say we have not sinned, we make him a liar,
and his word is not in us." 1 John 1:5-10

Nov 24th: LAST ONE! Chemo #16!!! WE DID IT!!! Here celebrating with my mom and as always my incredible nurse Jen!!!

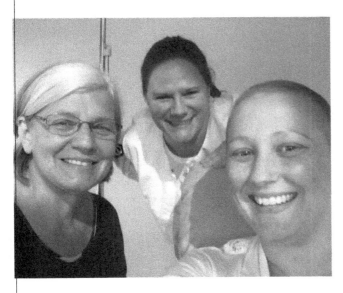

Mom and Dave have been with me every single step of the way. I can't imagine how I could have handled all this without their help! My mom has gone to most of the big Dr. appointments with me, helped with laundry (BIG JOB), helped with food and cleaning, and the most important help is playing and loving on my kids. She lives less than 5 minutes from me, and that has been such a blessing since she is able to swing by our house nearly everyday, sometimes multiple times a day. She helps when I'm weak, slow moving or need someone to talk to. We have always been the best of friends and I am so thankful she is my mom! I will keep you all posted as we get ready for the next phase -

Surgery. Lots of tests and appointments this month to prepare for the bilateral mastectomy, but for now I'm just happy to have part one of treatment done! Praise God, today is a great day!

"For everyone who has been born of God overcomes the world. And this is the victory that has overcome the world—our faith. Who is it that overcomes the world except the one who believes that Jesus is the Son of God?" 1 John 5: 4-5

MY FREE MONTH!

The below are my Facebook posts written during the beautiful month between my last chemo and surgery!

Dec 1st It's Tuesday and I am not going to chemo! Thankful for that! However, I am still going in for an appointment, an MRI. Then this Thursday the PET scan. These two tests I hope will confirm that the chemo did it's job and the cancer is gone. Regardless of what the test shows, I am thankful that God has carried me through these past 5 months and given me the strength to do much more than I'd thought possible. Even this week, reflecting on how much our family has to be thankful for, it's the very same reasons that we've always had, but it now seems even more clear. Little things like decorating for Christmas were always special, but now I can't help but get teary-eyed watching the kids and just being so thankful that I am here to enjoy their smiles and teach them more today. As I go into the MRI machine today, I will not be alone. God is with me. The lyrics of "Every Giant Will Fall" by Rend Collective, are on my heart today.

Dec 4th   I have very exciting news to share! I received my PET scan results this morning from Nurse Jen, and am happy to announce that I had a complete response to chemotherapy!!! This means the tumor is gone!!! Surgery should further decrease my chances of reoccurrence, so I am looking right at the finish line and excited to put this difficult time behind me. Praising God and reflecting on Psalm 118 today. The psalmist David says it perfectly! (See pg. 71)

Dec 22   It's been a little while since my last update, so I thought I'd let everyone know how I'm doing. GREAT! Very thankful to say that the last couple weeks I have really bounced back, I'm feeling healthy, and almost every side effect has disappeared. My energy is increasing daily and I am really enjoying that. I am able to cook and clean on my own. I don't need an afternoon nap and even make it till the kids bedtime most nights. I can sit on the floor and play games without pain, I was even able to do our walk to the local park this week. Many of the medical professionals I've seen in the past two weeks are astonished at how well I am doing, that my hair and skin coloring are returning so quickly, and that my overall wellbeing is so good. They've also said that I am tough, and have a high pain tolerance, I am thankful, but know that is a gift from God. He is my strength and my comfort. I still have one more week to enjoy fully before surgery. This month is a great break from the hard year we've had, and a good reminder of why this fight is so important. Daily life is beautiful, challenging yes, but beautiful. Take a moment to appreciate your health and look at your loved ones with true love and thankfulness.

"Cause me to hear Your loving kindness in the morning, For in You do I trust; Cause me to know the way in which I should walk, For I lift up my soul to You." Psalm 143:8 —

⁞ CHAPTER 8 ⁞
MIND OVER MATTER - SOUL OVER MIND

Like the daily life I had known before cancer, there were many good days and there were some rough, hard days too. During treatment that remained true, but the rough days felt more extreme. On some of those days, fatigue set in and I could not keep my eyes open through the day but when the house was finally dark and quiet and I should rest, the sleep wouldn't come. Some days, my bones ached so much that it hurt to put my feet on the ground. Some days the nausea would be so horrible that even a cup of water made me ill. Some days, the medications made thinking difficult and frustrating. Some days, I was so annoyed at my body that it made me annoyed with everything. Some days were rough. Really rough. It was in those times when my body and mind were just so exhausted, that my mind would start to wander. My thoughts would sometimes race or go very dark.

"But I call to God, and the LORD will save me. Evening and morning and at noon I utter my complaint and moan and he hears my voice" Psalm 55:16-17

I remember at my very first chemotherapy infusion, my nurse explained many symptoms that may arise and that depression can also become an issue for patients

> *Tip: If you feel like you need help, speak to your doctor. You may even want to speak about your medication options.*

and if I ever needed help to let them know. Being new to this and somewhat naive, I thought I was exempt. I knew I was in shock, but I didn't really think I'd struggle with depression.

Thankfully, I never felt that my rough days lasted long enough to need medication, but I do know that there were days that depression and anxiety tried to take hold of my mind.

"for God gave us a spirit not of fear but of power and love and self-control."

2 Timothy 1:7

Strangely, my anxiety often didn't seem directly related to being sick or even to treatment. It was not the usual fears of tests, scans, or surgeries. Mostly, it was my fear of not being the one to take care of my children. That fear would hit out of the blue, like a lightning bolt! Sometimes I'd have a bad dream, or it might be hearing someone else babysit the kids while I was resting, but mostly it was the times that my body and mind were just completely worn out.

I would start to panic. What would happen if I couldn't be the one to raise our children? How would my husband do everything? Would he move back to Ohio? Would he remarry? Would the kids be okay? I would panic and fret over things far beyond my control and become upset much too easily over news stories or world politics. I was afraid that I hadn't prepared the kids enough for what might lie ahead or what wars or persecution might come. Some days these fears would escalate way out of control!

On days like these, I felt disconnected and completely out of control. My soul knew to trust the Lord, but my mind would spin with worry, and my physical body was hurting and tired. Each piece tugging at me for attention. It was upsetting to feel this way. I knew that I wanted my soul to lead, but it was hard to silence the rest. In those times I needed to pray and to ask others to pray on my behalf too. I would pray for the Holy Spirit's comfort, for my soul and mind to be at peace. Then I would try to sleep. Thankfully, this anxiety was not a constant problem, but it did happen.

My mom and I can now look back and joke because after watching me wrestle with anxiety, we figured out a very simple physical remedy. I needed to treat myself like I would an infant! Seriously, when the depression and anxiety began I learned to ask myself the same questions that I asked when my newborns would cry. Is it: hunger, naptime, tummy trouble, or cuddle time? Not to sound patronizing, I'm completely serious! Once I figured this out, things did get a little easier. When my emotions started to unravel I would try to eat a little something, take a nap, or maybe a laxative. If those things didn't work I called the kids into bed to cuddle with me. Too simple? Maybe, but I'm telling you it helped. Sometimes I'd take a small dose of melatonin at night and go off into a deep rest, and by the next morning I usually felt myself again.

"Weeping may tarry for the night, but joy comes with the morning."

Psalm 30:5b

♡♡♡

I will try to provide more simple techniques that helped me when my head was clouded. On my good days these same things helped me keep a positive perspective.

This first action is so obvious, but I'm ashamed that it was not always the first thing to come to mind. I needed to pray! Like David did in Psalms, just cry out to the Lord. He has heard it all. He knows our hearts, so it's not like He will be surprised when we cry out that we feel afraid, worried, sad, etc... Amazing things happened when I went to the Lord. His presence brought clarity to situations, calmness to out-of-control emotions, and gave me His peace. Asking others to pray for us is humbling and encouraging too. I cannot describe my extreme emotions and gratitude, knowing that so many people cared enough for me to bring my troubles and needs to the Lord in prayer. I was so impacted by their acts of love and remembrance.

"The eyes of the LORD are toward the righteous and his ears toward their

cry. The face of the LORD is against those who do evil, to cut off the memory

of them from the earth. When the righteous cry for help, the LORD hears

and delivers them out of all their troubles. The LORD is near to the

brokenhearted and saves the crushed in spirit." Psalm 34: 15-18

I learned to surround myself with God's word. It might be a short verse on the refrigerator, a bookmark, a coffee mug, the cover of a day planner, etc... These are small things, but seeing the verses over and over again and really taking a moment to notice them helps commit the scripture to memory. They prompted me to think on good things even during mundane daily life. I also love quick, little devotional books with short passages that can be picked up and glanced through for a minute or an hour. Or the God's Promise-type books that list verses by the need or frame of mind. There are also great apps that can pop up and be a reminder of a bit of scripture to think on each day. Reading a Bible story to the children and asking them a few questions gets us all thinking about the Lord and about how important Jesus is for us and all the world. And, of course never letting the Bible collect dust! Opening it, reading it and really thinking about it, brought so much peace and clarity.

I'd sing loud! I've always loved music and singing in a choir or at church, but when I was sick for some reason I discovered how much I liked to lock myself away, (usually my bathroom) turn up the music, and sing loudly. Sometimes I'd think, "Lord, I hope this sounds good up there, please know that I love you." I'd sing, and I found that singing some of the same songs over and over, they became very personal. Those songs were sort of my own love letters to my Lord. Songs like those stay with you and sometimes I'd think of those songs as my anthem to get me through a specific milestone or week. I have a lot of favorite songs, but the one that always brings me joy and into a beautiful state of worship is "True Intimacy" by Rend Collective. When I first heard this song, I felt like someone had gathered up my thoughts and then let them out in a much more beautiful way than I could even attempted. Here are the lyrics:

True Intimacy
"Whatever I have; Whatever I hold;
There's nothing compares; To having You close
True intimacy; Is my desire
To catch Your whispers; To carry Your fire
You're my ambition; My destination
More than living; More than breathing
You're the reason; My heart's beating
There's nothing greater; Than knowing You
You unlock my joy; You waken my soul
Forever I'm Yours, God; Forever You're mine
A wonderful truth; That you are my life
You're my ambition; My soul's true mission
More than living; More than breathing
You're the reason; My heart's beating
So I'm giving; Freely yielding
You're the reason; My heart's beating
There's nothing greater than knowing You
Nothing greater than knowing You"

"The Lord is my strength and my shield; in him my heart trusts, and I am helped; my heart exults, and with my song I give thanks to him." Psalm 28:7

Calling out or singing the precious name of Jesus is so powerful! When I felt under attack spiritually, emotionally or physically, the name of Jesus was my battle cry. So many songs speak of this power because it is true! It could be a simple whisper, "Jesus, I need you." It could be a song, "Wonderful Grace of Jesus". His name has authority, and in His name devils are cast out, people are healed, believers are baptized, justified, and saved!

"Whatever you ask in my name, this I will do, that the Father may be glorified in the Son." John 14:13

A heart of gratitude is transforming. I found that writing thank you notes or jotting down positive experiences helped realign my thoughts. It is difficult to complain while giving thanks. Our prayers should be filled with thanksgiving, and so should our life. When I kept my eyes open and watching for the things to give thanks for, I was happily surprised that there is always something to be thankful for. My dad often says that everyday someone has it worse and someone has it better. This is true, and I know that even on my worst day there are still others that would have definitely traded me. There is always something or someone to be thankful for.

"Rejoice in the Lord always; again I will say, rejoice. Let your reasonableness be known to everyone. The Lord is at hand; do not be anxious about anything, but in everything by prayer and supplication with thanksgiving let your requests be made known to God. And the peace of God, which

surpasses all understanding, will guard your hearts and your minds in Christ Jesus. Finally, brothers, whatever is true, whatever is honorable, whatever is just, whatever is pure, whatever is lovely, whatever is commendable, if there is any excellence, if there is anything worthy of praise, think about these things. What you have learned and received and heard and seen in me—practice these things, and the God of peace will be with you." Philippians 4: 4-9

In Philippians 4:8 it lists what our minds should be filled with. If we keep looking for what is true, honorable, just, pure, lovely, commendable, excellent, and worthy of praise to think about, then our minds will be peaceful. Why is it so hard to do this? I think it is simply our human nature and this fallen sinful world that make it so easy to think about everything except these beautiful virtuous things. However, we have the gift of self-control to reign in these thoughts and to refocus on what is pleasing to God, and in turn it brings us comfort, joy and peace. I needed to think about good things.

I made myself do something fun. Made myself? I love to craft, but honestly, I was so tired that I really didn't have the desire to do much at all, even craft. The thought of pulling out supplies, making a mess, and having to clean up just kind of ruined the idea of even getting started. Finally, one day I thought that it had been too long since I did something just for fun, so I purchased myself some new paints. I did have fun, and I did make a mess and that was okay. I painted and my focus was just intently on the plaque I was designing for my daughters' room. I was in the moment and it was enjoyable and released some stress. I would enjoy thinking about the next piece that I could make, what I wanted it to say, what I wanted it to teach, and how it would make them feel. I ended up filling my daughters' wall with quotes and paintings that still make me smile every time I walk into their room.

I wrote love notes to my family. I felt like if the treatment worked, then these love notes would serve as a special reminder of how I felt about them in this brief window of time, almost like a time capsule. Or, if I wasn't able to get well, then I'd have said everything that I needed them to know about my love for them. My hospital gave us little stuffed bears for the kids to cuddle with when I was at the hospital and they had little pockets in the back where you could put notes. I made each child several little love letters and even laminated them so that they could always keep them. The notes said the things that made them special, the traits that I loved about them, my hopes for their future, and my prayers for them. Even though the kids are young, they loved those notes. They asked me to read them out loud to them over and over again many nights. I'm thankful that I did that and I'm not sure that I ever would have expressed things to them in that way had I not been sick. I have a feeling that those notes will have a far more lasting value than I had even hoped when I wrote them.

"I am the good shepherd.

The good shepherd lays down his life for the sheep." John 10:11

I think my favorite new habit became writing down "God sightings" in my journal. Years before I had cancer, our church in Ohio had an amazing VBS (Vacation Bible School) and on one big wall they hung a gigantic mural of green pastures. Each day teachers asked the children if there were examples in their life of "God sightings": times that they could feel God's presence, see His workmanship, or experience His teaching. This was so moving to me. Each day they posted these sweet little lambs up on the wall with the children's little testaments to God's personal connection to them. Some would have read statements like, "God made the stars", "God gave us food", "God taught us to love", "God created me", or "God sent us Jesus" etc.

The mural was also a beautiful visual of Christ being the shepherd over all these sweet children. I was sincerely inspired by this lesson even though it had been intended for all our small children.

As soon as I was diagnosed, the vivid memory of that mural with its green pasture, the lambs bearing witness to His glory, and Jesus our good shepherd all came to mind. This led to an inspiration that would sustain me throughout the coming year. It stirred me to write down all of my own "God sightings" as I could feel His presence, see His workmanship, experience his teachings, and (I added this last one) see His servants working as His hands. It was amazing to see how He was an integral part of this journey. I

> *Tip: Watch for all the ways God is present. Write them down and praise Him!*

was so thankful that He was carrying me and never left me alone.

My God sighting journal taught me how to keep watch for Him, and to notice all the incredible ways He was lovingly watching over me and our family. Had I not kept this journal, I believe I would have missed seeing many of his mercies and providences. I wonder how often moments have passed by with His gifts left unnoticed? Times when I should have stopped in awe, with pure gratitude and admiration.

Imagine in a world this immense, with so many little lambs, the good Shepherd is still keeping an eye on me! He cares about even little ol' me. Tenderly caring, and protecting me. I am humbled at the thought. How great and amazing is our God!

"fear not, for I am with you; be not dismayed, for I am your God; I will strengthen you, I will help you, I will uphold you with my righteous right hand." Isaiah 41:10

: CHAPTER 9 :
PAUL POINTS UP TO JESUS

It's just not fair! Why did this happen to me? Cancer never feels fair, but it really is unbiased. Cancer doesn't limit whom it chooses. It strikes the wealthy and the poor, men and women, every personality, the old and the young. Cancer is not picky. The unfair part of cancer is the fact that it even exists. I think that is why every cancer patient feels it's unfair. It was easy to become bitter and sad about the whole situation, but I knew that was not the attitude God desired of me.

I knew that the Holy Spirit gives beautiful gifts of love, joy, peace, patience, kindness, goodness, faithfulness, gentleness and self-control. Not of bitterness nor sadness!

How was I to be joyful during cancer?

While reading Philippians, I kept reading the Apostle Paul talk of joy and I knew in my heart that I shared that same joy, but I was losing perspective being so entrenched with the physical burdens of illness. So I really started thinking about Paul and what I have in common with him.

Before I can look at what we have in common, let's briefly look at his testimony. In his early life, Paul was known as Saul, always a passionate man full of zeal. But before knowing Jesus, he was cruel and ruthless against Christians. He believed that those working in the name of Jesus were heretics and his passion was to find them and punish them.

"But Saul was ravaging the church, and entering house after house, he dragged off men and women and committed them to prison." Acts 8:3

Saul had come to his peak of vengeance and was just about to set out on his personal mission to gather up and quiet all of Jesus' followers when his life was completely changed. As he set out on his journey, he was caught up in a bright light from heaven. He fell to the ground and heard Jesus voice saying, "Saul, Saul, why are you persecuting me?" Saul asks, "Who are you Lord?" and Jesus answers him, "I am Jesus, whom you are persecuting". Jesus then gave Saul instructions on where to go, and from that life-changing moment, Saul obeyed the Lord. Only our Lord could, in a moment turn an enemy into a follower! Saul obeyed, and through prayer in Jesus' name he was baptized and received the Holy Spirit. Below is Paul's testimony directly from the book of Acts 9:

"But Saul, still breathing threats and murder against the disciples of the Lord, went to the high priest and asked him for letters to the synagogues at Damascus, so that if he found any belonging to the Way, men or women, he might bring them bound to Jerusalem. Now as he went on his way, he approached Damascus, and suddenly a light from heaven shone around him. And falling to the ground, he heard a voice saying to him, "Saul, Saul, why are you persecuting me?" And he said, "Who are you, Lord?" And he said, "I am Jesus, whom you are persecuting. But rise and enter the city, and you will be told what you are to do." The men who were traveling with him stood speechless, hearing the voice but seeing no one. Saul rose from the ground, and although his eyes were opened, he saw nothing. So they led him by the hand and brought him into Damascus. And for three days he was without sight, and neither ate nor drank. Now there was a disciple at Damascus named Ananias. The Lord said to him in a vision, "Ananias." And he said, "Here I am, Lord." And the Lord said to him, "Rise and go to the street called Straight, and at the house of Judas look for a man of Tarsus named Saul, for behold, he is praying, and he has seen in a vision a man named Ananias come in and lay his hands on him so that he might regain his sight." But Ananias answered, "Lord, I have heard from many about this man, how much evil he has done to your saints at Jerusalem. And here he has authority from the chief priests to bind all who call on your name." But the Lord said to him, "Go, for he is a chosen instrument of mine to carry my name before the Gentiles and kings and the children of Israel. For I will show him how much he must suffer for the sake of my name." So Ananias departed and entered the house. And laying his hands on him he said, "Brother Saul, the Lord Jesus who appeared to you on the road by which you came has sent me so that you may regain your sight and be filled with the Holy Spirit." And immediately something like scales fell from his eyes, and he regained his sight. Then he rose and was baptized; and taking food, he was strengthened."

Acts 9: 1-19

Did Paul now have a picture-perfect life? Did he go home and relax in joy knowing that he was saved? He no longer needed to fight Christians. He had become one! Was his job done? Did he turn to creature comforts like so many in this world do, looking to find happiness in a quiet, easy life? Turn to hobbies, pleasures or doing only what made him happy? No, quite the opposite. His new life as Paul was difficult, painful, and selfless, yet he was still one of the most joyful people I've ever learned about. So, how is he so different than so many people who seek joy?

I recall trying to show my youngest daughter a hummingbird hovering way up in the branches of a tall tree and she could not see it. I tried describing it, saying "Honey, look up, even higher. Crouch down from over here." It wasn't until I physically took her face in my hands and directed her eyes up at the hummingbird. Then I pointed up with my arm outstretched and said, "See it's right there, up in front of us!" This is like what Paul did for me! He redirected my eyesight and fixed my eyes upon our common ground, which is Jesus Christ, our Lord and Savior

If I try to find joy in this world, nothing remains the same or is reliable. However, if my joy rests solely in Jesus Christ, it is forever.

"Jesus Christ is the same yesterday and today and forever."

Hebrews 13:8

Apostle Paul's testimony is drastically different than mine, but after his conversion we began to have some things in common, mostly our joy in Christ! My joy was rooted in the gift that God gave through His son Jesus Christ and what He has done for me. What happened generations ago is not just some part of history, it is MY HISTORY! It is part of my testimony, and it is the part of my life that began before I even took my first breath. Once I claimed Jesus as part of my own life story, my testimony and witness became much more powerful, because in the name of Jesus is power! What did Jesus do in my life? Jesus came to Earth in the flesh. He taught me by word and example. He explained the wonders of heaven and the plan of salvation. He lived a life of servant-hood and obedience. And, though He lived an innocent life, He willingly sacrificed Himself to a brutal physical death at the cross, shedding His pure innocent blood to cover my sins! This is part of my life story. Jesus is my hero. Paul knows that Jesus is part of his own life story too. We share this hero, Jesus! Paul writes,

"Have this mind among yourselves, which is yours in Christ Jesus, who, though he was in the form of God, did not count equality with God a thing to be grasped, but emptied himself, by taking the form of a servant, being

born in the likeness of men. And being found in human form, he humbled himself by becoming obedient to the point of death, even death on a cross. Therefore God has highly exalted him and bestowed on him the name that is above every name, so that at the name of Jesus every knee should bow, in heaven and on earth and under the earth, and every tongue confess that Jesus Christ is Lord, to the glory of God the Father." Philippians 2: 5-11

However, that is not all! My joy doesn't only rest in the past, but it is anchored to my hope in the future I have through Jesus. Paul and I will share in that future as it is promised. Christ will return for us. He will know us and make us citizens of His heavenly city! Jesus said:

"My sheep hear my voice, and I know them, and they follow me. I give them eternal life, and they will never perish, and no one will snatch them out of my hand. My Father, who has given them to me, is greater than all, and no one is able to snatch them out of the Father's hand.

I and the Father are one." John 10:27-30

Thinking of my history in Jesus and my future in Him, how can I not be full of joy? How can my soul not rejoice in thankfulness? This is the true joy apostle Paul writes so much about.

"Rejoice in the Lord always; again I will say, rejoice." Philippians 4:4

Even though Paul faced extreme difficulty while on Earth; being beaten, imprisoned, under house arrest and even survived being stoned, I don't read of any complaint in his letters. He viewed every affliction, and every suffering as an opportunity to further the gospel and share his history and future in Christ with everyone. What a high standard! I know I complained about my own troubles and next to so many people in the Bible, my suffering cannot begin to be compared. I sometimes needed to express my sorrows but this put it in a new perspective. I hoped that my affliction might be used in some way to bring God glory. Like Paul, I started looking as those moments as opportunities to spread the gospel. Every patient, nurse, and Facebook friend was someone with whom I could share The Word. Even if it was only one scripture verse at a time, I wanted to find joy in furthering the gospel like Paul did. I admire Paul's boldness, because sharing our faith takes courage!

I remember the excitement I felt when I received a message from a friend who said, "I prayed for you even though I don't normally pray." I was brought to tears, and thought that had I not been sick, this person might not have prayed, might not have knocked at God's door, and though I may never know what comes of it, I am so thankful that even one prayer was offered because of my illness. I trust that the Lord used my trial for much more good than I will ever know.

"Count it all joy, my brothers, when you meet trials of various kinds, for you know that the testing of your faith produces steadfastness.

And let steadfastness have its full effect,

that you may be perfect and complete, lacking in nothing."

James 1:2-4

I sometimes talked to my friends and family about having an unfair advantage compared to other patients. It was true - Paul and I both had an advantage! While facing even the hardest days or the most physically difficult situations, our eyes could stay fixed on Jesus. The joy that Jesus gives outweighs every sorrow and every burden. The joy He gives is constant no matter what emotion or feeling the day brings. When we acknowledge Christ as our personal Savior, His power is above all else! Christ is our power and our joy!

"For I consider that the sufferings of this present time are not worth

comparing with the glory that is to be revealed to us."

Romans 8:18

: CHAPTER 10 :
JUST CUT THEM OFF!

G oing into treatment, I really didn't know anything about mastectomies. I thought there was one option; to "cut them off". Little did I know that there are numerous types of surgery options, and I had to make some decisions regarding this part of my treatment plan. I was surprised by how overwhelming all of the information felt, and how difficult it was to sift through the different options to figure out what was actually my choice verses a doctor's decision. I became very thankful that up to this point in treatment, I hadn't had much role in decision making; the doctor advised a plan and I went with it.

For many breast cancer patients a mastectomy or lumpectomy comes quickly after being diagnosed, and before chemotherapy to prevent the cancer from spreading. This is not the current recommendation for treating my Triple-Negative Breast Cancer. In this specific type of breast cancer, it is common to have chemotherapy first because it is such a fast-spreading, fast-growing cancer and can sometimes be resistant to chemotherapy or have metastasized. For these reasons, some doctors opt to measure the tumor and begin chemotherapy and scan to measure again later, making sure that the cancer is responding to the chemotherapy. This is significant because if the cancer has spread any cells to other areas of the body, the doctors want to be sure the chemotherapy is effectively destroying all cancer cells throughout the body. Thankfully for me, the chemotherapy was effective and after treatment my tumor was nearly non-existent! During chemotherapy, and in the months leading up to my mastectomy, I had time to plan and choose what my surgery would entail. I needed to choose both my oncology surgeon and plastic surgeon for reconstruction.

My oncologist was a huge help and referred me to an oncology surgeon, who is an exceptional surgeon with an amazing bedside manner. On our first meeting she walked me through options and gave me a wealth of much-needed information. I had the options of a lumpectomy, a one-sided mastectomy, or a full bilateral mastectomy. Given my specific case, she helped me to make the hard decision of going for the full-bilateral mastectomy. She then told me that I have even more options about the appearance and physical reconstruction, but need to choose a plastic surgeon to make those decisions.

Tip: When making these decision look to your doctor to educates you on the options and how it may affect your after-care treatment, possible reoccurrence risks, radiation therapy and the overall appearance. All of these factor will contribute to the decision you come to with your doctor.

I went to three plastic surgeons for consultations and guidance. I found the process of choosing the right reconstruction very difficult and emotional. Even the initial consultation with each plastic surgeon proved taxing on my emotions and self-esteem. I would need to get undressed for each of their assessments and detailed measurements. I recall standing in one office specifically feeling so vulnerable and broken. I remember thinking of my body with such disgust. Here I am, at a place where women go to look like dolls and find physical perfection! Instead, I'm here with no hair, eyebrows or lashes, a chubby belly, stretch marks and cancerous breasts that need removed. I felt so out of place. I don't usually care much about my appearance, but that day I wished the doctor could just transplant me to a completely new body! At that moment I despised my own body. I left that appointment in tears. I did not have peace at that office and I wasn't going back. Thankfully, I did find that one of the three doctors did make me feel at ease and normal. She proved to be not only a good choice, but in the end I know she was the best choice for me.

Once I knew that I'd selected my plastic surgeon, she helped me look at my choices for reconstruction. I was not a candidate for all options, narrowing it down a bit. I chose the surgery I felt most comfortable with and seemed to make the most sense for my specific situation. I chose an immediate, nipple-sparing, direct-to-implant with gummies, complete mastectomy. Yes, there is quite a lot of information in that description. Going into surgery that morning, I did not know if my choice was even possible, being dependent on my pathology report, taken *during* the mastectomy for immediate analysis. My plastic surgeon would make the final decision for me *during* surgery, based on the pathology report and my skin's viability. I had to trust my doctor to make the best call for me. Thankfully, my results were all good and it allowed my doctor to perform my first choice in reconstruction options.

"Therefore do not be anxious about tomorrow, for tomorrow will be anxious for itself. Sufficient for the day is its own trouble."

Matthew 6:34

♡♡♡

My Surgery Experience

I completed chemotherapy five weeks before surgery. This gave me a beautiful window of time to get as healthy as possible and really savor my time with my family! I could not have asked for better timing as Christmas was during that break. Having those weeks to prepare for surgery also put me at an advantage for recovery since I was able to prepare everything ahead of time. I planned and set up my recover area just the way I liked it. I am very thankful for this because I did experience complications with recovery and it took a bit longer than I had anticipated.

The day before surgery I took my kids over to Deb's house. She is a life-long friend and I knew she would take excellent care of them while I was at the hospital and for the first few days of recovery. I wanted them to be with her, away from the stresses that Dave and my mom would be under. I didn't want them to worry or overhear phone calls or be juggled by babysitters as Dave went back and forth from the hospital. This worked out really well; the kids felt like this was a special vacation and were looking forward to spending a few days there. Deb even planned a couple play dates with their friends from church to fill their time with fun and excitement. I dropped them off with their love notes and humongous hugs, knowing that the next time I saw them those hugs would hurt. I walked out her door with tears in my eyes, but the kids were happy and safe and that put me at ease.

From there, I went to the hospital to have dye injected through the nipple to help my surgeon examine and remove my sentinel lymph node during my mastectomy the next day. My doctor had warned me that the injections are quite uncomfortable and that I could use my numbing EMLA cream before arriving to help numb the area. The doctor who gave me this injection was pleasantly surprised and told me most doctors don't tell the patients about the cream and it really is helpful. I went home without pain and tried to get a good night's sleep.

The morning of surgery I went in about two hours early for pre-op. This was my first planned surgery and I was surprised how quickly the time passed moving from registration, to changing, to receiving the IV, and finally meeting the anesthesiologist. Thankfully, I was given medication through the IV to relax me and I don't even remember them strolling me into the hallway. It really worked that fast!

When I woke up after surgery, the room was spinning and my nurses saw my trouble before I could even utter a word. They quickly gave me an injection and cool cloths to calm the nausea. While I did get sick for a little while, they were able to get the nausea under control with a scopolamine patch behind my ear. It was my first experience with patches and now I request them before any surgery. Once the nausea subsided, they strolled me up to my hospital room. I remember feeling barely awake and like there was a very heavy weight over my chest. I was not in sharp pain at all. I was advised to start getting up and walking as soon as possible after surgery, so though it was difficult, I did stand up and use the bathroom that same day. By the next day, I was able to make a slow, short lap around the hospital floor. I remember how strange my body felt; as though I was pieced together. Some areas were sore, some numb, and other parts extremely heavy. I was so very proud of myself for walking, and while it was difficult, I was never in extreme pain. The pain medication always worked for me and I would describe the experience more like an odd discomfort that comes from a heaviness and inability to move around. My body was weak, numb, and heavy - unlike anything I had known, yet after only 1 day, I was

> *Tip: Movement actually aids healing and prevents other complications!*

able to go home. I remember feeling queasy in the car and extremely tired. I slept a lot for the next few days.

Overall, my mastectomy was a success. All of the breast tissue was removed along with the tiny little speck of cancer that was remaining after chemotherapy, (so small it had not even been detected on the scans) and thankfully my lymph nodes were also clear. I was thrilled with that news and happy to consider myself to be cancer-free!

Once I was at home, my recovery did not take the expected path. Overall, recovery was very slow and difficult, but I believe that the first few days at home were fairly similar to what most mastectomy patience experience.

I was blessed to have my husband Dave, my mom and my sister-in-law Adrienne, all available to help take care of me and the children. Their help was critical, because I could barely keep my eyes open and was incredibly dependent on others for everything. The pain pill medication was not as effective as the hospital IV medication, but I still don't recall ever being in unbearable pain, just sore and so very tired. I did need someone right beside me for the first few days when I was standing because I did feel very faint, and nearly fell down a couple of times. Aside from helping me get up and walking, they also tracked my medications, kept small portions of food available, and were literally there for my every need.

I am a modest person and it was very difficult to allow them to help me to the bathroom, into the shower and then to get dressed. Though I wished I could have done it on my own, that was simply impossible. I was dizzy, weak, and in pain, so I knew that it would actually be dangerous to attempt anything on my own.

It was also nice to have their help with opening up all of the bandages and gauze, laying them carefully out in order so that changing out the old ones wasn't too difficult. Adrienne also took care of emptying and measuring my drains for the first few days. She was a nurse and this was something she did quickly and she made it look simple.

I was thankful for all of the help, because just getting out of a chair at that point was hard work. Each day I did get a little bit stronger and a tiny bit more independent, but my body encountered some extreme problems healing.

Those unexpected problems created many delays in recovery, but I will explain that in more detail throughout the chapter describing my next unusual experience inside the hyperbaric therapy chamber.

♡♡♡

Practical Advice to Prepare for Recovery

-Support:

You will need someone with you when you leave the hospital and you should have someone at home to help you get up and down, bring you food and medication for the first few days. I was blessed to have my amazing sister-in-law, Adrienne, stay with us. She is also a nurse, so I really could not have been in better hands. .

> *Tip: If you don't have someone able to assist you with medical tasks, like emptying your drains, ask your surgeon if there is a nursing service that can come and help you in the days following surgery.*

-A comfortable area to rest:

I borrowed my parents' electric recliner and it was absolutely perfect. The power buttons made gentle reclining and getting up much easier. I could not get into my tall bed for quite a while, and the recliner was in eyesight of our tv which helped pass the time. I watched a lot of Netflix. I also had a table on each side to keep my care items (drink, remote, tissues, phone, etc.) easily accessible. I had lymph node removal on my right so I could not reach with my right arm, but it was still nice to keep everything close by. I kept a lap tray next to the recliner for my meals and I even hung my clipboard on the wall below my kids' pictures so we could easily mark down medications and drainage information. Other helpful items were the laptop and CD player because music was healing and therapeutic for me.

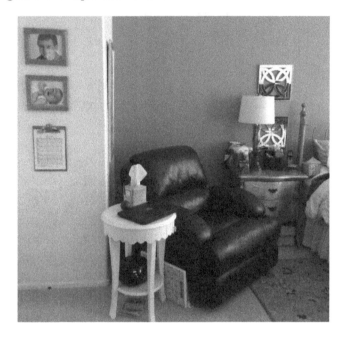

-Button front shirts and pajamas:

It will be a while before you can comfortably pull anything up over your head. They should be a size larger than you normally wear to accommodate swelling, bandages, and tubes. Have a few so that you are not stuck needing laundry done every day.

-Xeroform , medical pads, and gauze:

You will likely need dry sterile gauze as well as medicated gauze called Xeroform to help with healing. It is put over the sutures, and then medical pads are layered next to help absorb and protect. Your plastic surgeon should recommend or order the quantities you need.

-Prescriptions:

Prefill medications, and keep a notepad and pen handy to log what time each prescription was taken. I was very groggy and could not remember anything so writing down the times was critical.

-Extra Pillows:

I had one ready in the car for the ride home from the hospital, and kept several extras around my recovery area. I found that I could sleep better with a pillow on each side of me so I wouldn't twist or roll even an inch in my sleep. I also liked one across my chest area when I was sitting, the extra cushion and protection was comforting. While I was still stitched and healing, a pillow in front of me served as a deterrent from hugs. Everyone wanted to hug me and make me feel better (especially the kids), but until I was ready for hugs I learned to keep the pillow nearby so it would remind them that I was not yet ready. I was given a couple medium-sized heart shaped pillows and they were very nice for under the arms, because for the first few days everything is still very sensitive and tender.

-Mastectomy bras and drainage apron or pockets:

The doctor can often prescribe these as part of your covered medical supplies. These are soft, front-closing bras that stretch to accommodate swelling and bandages. Mine also came with pockets to hold pads in case you need the volume added until future reconstruction. They also supplied me with drain pockets that hold the drains and Velcro up to the bra. I was also supplied with a drain apron and shower accessory to help with drain tubes. I had two drain tubes post-surgery, but some have up to four. It felt more comfortable with the bulb at the ends secured in a drain apron or up inside my shirt. The gravity would pull at my incision site if they were just hanging down at my sides. When I showered, it helped to use a lanyard around my neck to hold up the drain tubes so they were not pulling down.

-A chart to track the drainage:

The hospital supplied a chart. I kept it on a clipboard near my chair to track and clean my drain tubes without having to stand up. The doctor used these records to determine when I could have the tubes come out. I expected to have the drains for up to a week, but only had to keep them for about 4 days. That's not too long at all, but I sure was very happy to see them go.

-Rubbing alcohol wipes:

The wipes are handy to clean the drain tubes and your hands after emptying the drains out.

Below are my Facebook posts from the day of surgery
and all the way through my long recovery.

Dec 30th Surgery is today.
Praying the Lord will be my strength and my
comfort through both the surgery and recovery.
That He would guide the doctors with wisdom to do
what is best and right for me. And that the
pathologies will confirm that I am cancer free.
Praying for peace with whatever these next
hours/days hold and that my joy and appreciation
can be felt by everyone I meet here at Virginia G
Piper! Thank you
all for your love
and prayers!

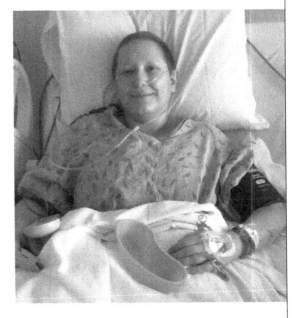

Dec 30th

(Posted by Dave)

God is good.
Successful
surgery, updates
to come.
Thank you all for
your prayers and support! -d

Dec 31st: (Posted by Dave)

Adrienne arrived from Ohio today in time to help get Laura situated here at home. Thanks again to those praying and helping. Knowing we can never repay you all for your selfless support, in so many ways, is reminiscent of Laura and my salvation through Jesus Christ; all more than we could describe, or have foreseen or earned...and can't ever fully grasp even after it has been received.

Each note, prayer, letter, call or message serves as a small window through which we have glimpses into seeing unconditional love shared with us through trials, just as our Father offers love through Jesus' sacrifice. I've read Laura each of your posts yesterday and she was thankful for them, and I'm certain she'll be re-reading them herself again for encouragement throughout the coming days.

I'm certain she'll be updating statuses early in the new year, so be on the lookout...as usual, her posts will end with grace and class. Mine just end with '-d'. May God bless you all with peace, joy and comfort in 2016, and may His glory and praise be in our hearts no matter what the New Year brings. And for whatever 2016 will bring us, we will bring His praise. -d

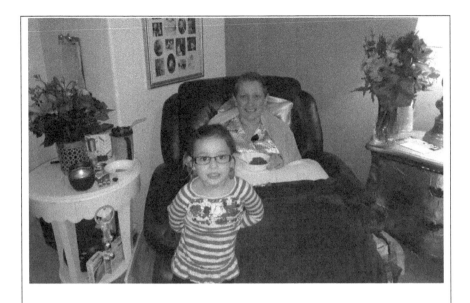

January 7th

What a week! Started with a bilateral Mastectomy and immediate reconstruction! (Praise God that is what I was hoping for) The week of recovery is not what I pictured. I thought I'd be snuggled up in my chair watching Netflix laughing with Adrienne. Instead it has been a very busy week seeing four doctors and undergoing hyperbaric chamber treatments daily

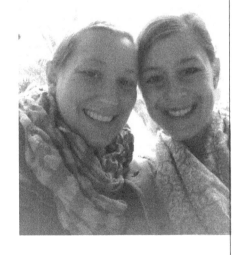

to help the blood flow in my skin. There have been many tears, pain, moments of confusion and extreme exhaustion BUT overall everything is going very well! The surgery revealed that there was less than 1 millimeter of cancer remaining this reassures me that the bilateral mastectomy was the best choice ever! This also means no radiation is needed!!! I thank God for all the people helping with the kids and for helping me. My Adrienne really has been the best medicine and I thank God for her. My loving Dave and devoted parents are amongst the greatest gifts God has ever given me! Most of all the joy of the Lord is my strength!!!!

January 14th

Gotta love cousins!!! Jackie was out taking care of me again. And who trained her??? Another beautiful and kind cousin, Denise! I have amazing family! Thanks for doing the dirty work girls!!!!

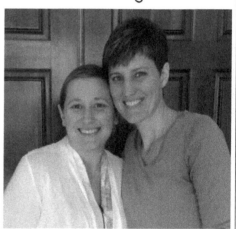

Jan 18th

Health update. Recovery from my Mastectomy has been pretty slow, and my skin is having difficulty healing. So today the doctor decided that to improve my skins health and prevent further complications I will need another minor surgery tomorrow (Tuesday). I'll be arriving at noon and should be in recovery by 3:00. I appreciate your prayers!

Jan 25th

It has been over 3 weeks of recovery, and it has possibly been the hardest time of my life. Recovery has not been easy and we've faced some struggles, but as with everything there is always much to be

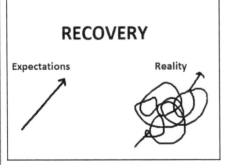

thankful for. Today I met again with my surgeon and she is pleased with the current status from Tuesdays minor surgery.

She said she is hopeful that we are now headed in the right direction. -If- my incisions continue to heal properly than I may get to have the stitches out next Monday, and -if- the blood flow in my skin continues to improve than I may only have 7 more hyperbaric treatments to go. This is a lot to hope for and a lot to pray for. I am ready to move forward. I am thankful to say that both my sinus infection and pneumonia are improving greatly which makes my time in the hyperbaric much more tolerable, and hopefully now I will be getting even more oxygen into my lungs/blood/skin. This should help for all around improved healing. My flexibility has really improved in the last couple days and my energy has made a few short appearances so I can trust that day by day I am getting stronger. I am continuously moved to tears by the amount of love and support I am surrounded by. I am blessed so much by all of the people in my life. I often feel guilty because of how good I have it by comparison to so many other patients I see. Thank you all for making a hard time into something good, by showing me beauty everyday in all the ways you love me and the family. The cards, texts, food, babysitting etc.... I cannot express my thanks fully enough!

Feb 1st: Well today's appointment didn't go as I'd hoped for. Instead of getting my stitches removed they were replaced and will come out in three weeks. I will continue hyperbaric for another 2 1/2 weeks. My skin is improving, just very slowly. This is a common problem after chemotherapy, my skin is just still very weak. At least there is progress and we are going in the right direction.

I am thankful for a great Dr who I trust! God bless all those in the medical field, it is a tough line of work! Those that have the talent and the people skills are a gift and I truly appreciate them!

Feb 17 Today is my 30th and final hyperbaric treatment here at Osborn. I was almost afraid to get excited about this until yesterday when I really believed it was the end!! Now I am overjoyed! Even though I am still all stitched up (on my 6th set of stitches, boo!), that is all that remains and then I can really move on. This is all nearly a memory! This recovery has been so hard, but today I reflect on one of the biggest blessings of cancer, and that is all the new people I've met! I have had so many great conversations with so many people that I would have otherwise never met. The doctors, nurses, chemo patients, cancer survivors, radiation patients, diabetic amputees, many of their friends and family

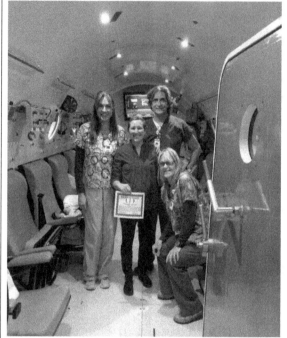 members in the waiting rooms, strangers that see me and recognize the distinctive marks of battling cancer and want to share their personal experiences....

I've met so many people and I feel like I've learned a little from every single one! There are many many more faithful God loving people out there than I thought and that gives me lots of hope for my children in a world that often feels quite sad. And those that don't have that same Faith or Joy, well I hope I was able to cheer and encourage some of them. I tried to show kindness to everyone I met and my heart was full because of their kindness toward me.

God has been my comfort and strength and I am

thankful that He has guided me through this valley showing me the beauty with each step.

A Psalm of David. Psalm 23 "The Lord is my shepherd; I shall not want. He makes me lie down in green pastures. He leads me beside still waters. He restores my soul. He leads me in paths of righteousness for his name's sake. Even though I walk through the valley of the shadow of death, I will fear no evil, for you are with me; your rod and your staff, they comfort me. You prepare a table before me in the presence of my enemies; you anoint my head with oil; my cup overflows. Surely goodness and mercy shall follow me all the days of my life, and I shall dwell in the house of the Lord forever."

Note: I had two surgeries in the months following my mastectomy. Both were necessary to remove necrotic tissue "dead skin" that did not have blood flow.

Feb 28 (Posted by Dave) Laura has just been taken into surgery. Certainly a busy day in the OR, with multiple urgent cases bumping her back throughout the day, who could also use our prayers today. And God will be praised. Thanks again for all of your prayers and support, and I'll be sure to post an update on her condition later this evening. -d

⦂CHAPTER 11⦂
DIVING DEEP IN HYPERBARIC

I was resting in my electric powered recliner, pain medications doing their work, and the peace of mind that the cancer had been surgically removed and was no longer in my body. I was so excited, so ready to move forward and wave a hearty goodbye to cancer. Unfortunately it wasn't that simple.

At my very first post-surgical follow-up appointment the plastic surgeon already saw that things were not going according to plan. My skin was red and irritated, some skin was turning too black, and my doctor knew that my blood flow was not ideally flowing all throughout the wound. It was early on, but my doctor wisely prescribed hyperbaric oxygen therapy. I had never heard of this but was ready to follow her instructions. I never could have anticipated just how life-changing this experience would end up being for me.

Hyperbaric oxygen therapy is breathing pure oxygen while inside a pressurized tube (individual) or a submarine-type room (group). It is the same technique used for scuba divers with a condition called "the bends" (decompression sickness). It can be used to heal serious infections, air bubbles in blood vessels, and wounds that won't heal; often as a result of diabetes or radiation burns. The therapy works by increasing air pressure on the body up to three times higher than normal, causing the lungs to take in more oxygen than normally possible. The blood is then packed full of oxygen to deliver all throughout the body. This oxygen helps fight bacteria and stimulate growth factor and stem cells which provide significant healing. It is an amazing science to learn about and I loved hearing the nurses describe it to each new patient.

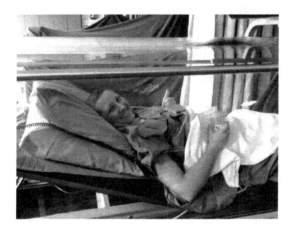

The first few therapy sessions were at a hospital using only individual dive chambers. These are clear acrylic chambers with a bed that rolls into them. Picture Snow White's coffin. That's what it looked like to me. They would give me a sippy-cup to help me clear my ears while they were pressurizing the chamber. It is much like going up.. up.. up.. in an airplane and having your ears pop, or in the times when the pressure was even more noticeably intense, it would feel like diving down and holding myself at the bottom of a 10 foot swimming pool. I never had much trouble getting my ears pressurized when sipping on water and tugging at my ears in the individual chamber. After a few treatments we realized that the therapy was better-covered by our insurance at a different hospital, primarily using the large submarine-style chamber. This was a completely different experience.

Each day, people would board the submarine wearing either hospital scrubs or 100% cotton clothing to ensure nothing was flammable. There could be no metal (no zippers, buttons, watches, etc.). No lotions or gels. Absolutely nothing that could be flammable or cause a spark to risk combustion. Now that's a sobering thought when you're trapped in a submarine with strangers. I just hoped they were all rule-followers like me!

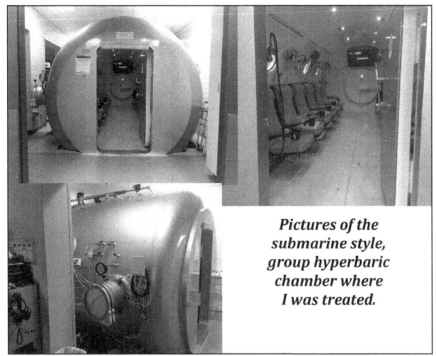

*Pictures of the
submarine style,
group hyperbaric
chamber where
I was treated.*

The submarine could hold approximately twelve people and there was always a nurse on board. As we entered the submarine two nurses lowered an elastic neck collar down over our heads and asked us to choose a seat. When everyone was seated and ready they would seal the door closed and a hissing sound would begin. This was the sound of pressurization. At this point, our nurse would walk around passing out a small cup of water and a straw, a piece of chewing gum, and a tissue. My first day in the submarine I thought it was out of courtesy, but these were actually essential tools for popping ears, clearing noses, and getting us pressurized.

Once we hit our specific dive level, the patients would put big headphones over their ears and the nurse would come around attaching a plastic helmet to our neck collars over our heads for an air-tight fit. We looked a bit like astronauts at sea. I found us all looking rather hysterical, but tried to hide my amusement. The nurse then quickly connected the input and output for our pure, oxygenated air. She also connected our headphone cable to a connector. A television located at the front of the sub would turn on and today's 2 hour featured film would begin playing, like it or not. I also learned that I am not at all a movie connoisseur and am an incredibly picky person. Seeing over 30 movies over the course of therapy, there were only about 5 I'd even consider watching again. Many were too scary or too sad, and once the helmet was on, I couldn't even wipe away the tears. Regardless of the movie, when we were geared up and breathing that precious pure oxygen, we were all set to begin healing.

I continued on in this large submarine every weekday for thirty consecutive days. In total this was six weeks of side-by-side interactions with three rotating nurses and many fascinating patients who came and went. My plastic surgeon had initially estimated that I'd have about ten days of treatment, but again recovery didn't go as expected. My body at this point was incredibly weak, so weak in fact that I had contracted pneumonia and my skin didn't want to hold any stitches. There were many contributing factors so it was impossible to know exactly why this was happening, but it was probably because I had just finished chemotherapy and was still recovering. Or perhaps in part because of my latex allergy, or because I've been borderline diabetic in the past. We also discovered that I have difficult skin that does not like to heal, having had a difficult time healing with this surgery and following my caesarian section five years earlier. At that time doctors blamed my slow healing on having the cold virus. I was in the hospital for a week after my daughter's birth and I never expected this would be a problem I'd ever face again. Again, facing the same skin challenges, it became obvious that I have very sensitive and delicate skin. And while the doctor explained that all of these factors may contribute, most of all it was the chemotherapy that made my skin so thin and weak. The healing was going very, very slowly.

Hyperbaric therapy is an amazing technology that does so much good and can be so incredibly healing, but it is not without downsides. It also causes extreme fatigue. Between my body healing from surgery, chemotherapy and pneumonia, still being on quite a lot of medication and now the added fatigue of hyperbaric therapy, I ended up completely exhausted and in a sort of foggy reality. The first weeks of hyperbaric, I remember as though it were all a dream.

My sister-in-law Adrienne often brings to mind the memory of us singing to one of my favorite songs on our drive home from hyperbaric that first week. I vaguely remember it and it doesn't even feel real. If she didn't insist, I would've thought it was all just a dream.

After the first ten days of hyperbaric we could tell that it was helping the blood flow, but my stitches still wouldn't stay in. Each time the stitches would loosen up, leaving a gap in my wound or even worse, the thread would just bury themselves right down through the skin. We tried a few types of thread, techniques, and different healing medications, but this cycle continued. So every few days I would be back in my plastic surgeons' out-patient surgical room and we would replace the stitches again. This happened many times and it was frustrating every time, to have stitches put in and the closure be good and tight, hoping that this was the last time. I was hoping that I wouldn't have to go through this again, and feeling like I'm starting all over with recovery. It was a discouraging cycle. I thought this was a normal complication, but over time I knew that this was very unusual. I was thankful that I trusted my doctor and she was patient and vigilantly watched over my recovery.

All along I continued on my daily schedule with hyperbaric. As I got stronger and more accustomed to the very unique hyperbaric therapy routine, I actually felt at home in the submarine. I realized that I could serve a purpose in the submarine and, strangely enough, this realization changed my whole perspective going in each day.

Most of the people I met in hyperbaric were in one of three categories, all quite different than my own. One group was of those recovering from a terrible car crash; they were extremely injured and probably had crushed bones and multiple surgeries to repair their body. They were in desperate, immediate need of healing. The second group was the most common patient, the diabetics. Often these were older men who had their toes amputated or were missing a foot or a leg. For many of them, this was their last hope for not losing the next limb. This was a continual battle and something that became a large part of their life. Finally, there were the cancer patients, many of which had just finished radiation and their skin was dry, tender and burned. They were recovering, tired, and needed healing. I could relate with these patients the best, though I had never been through their experience either. I never met anyone else like me, with my history or a similar story, but we were all there to heal.

Within my first week of submarine dives there was a man who was very upset and didn't like the idea of being stuck in a submarine or having his head in a plastic helmet. He was rather difficult for the nurse, and I remember feeling somewhat scared at first, just hoping he wasn't going to throw a fit or cause a big problem. But as I sat across from him in the submarine, I could see his sadness. So I began to talk to him. I asked "Have you ever done this before?" and he had a lot! From there he wanted to tell me his story. He told me all he's been through and how sick and how painful his life was. He just needed some compassionate ears to hear him and show a little bit of kindness. After he'd expressed his frustration and sadness he calmed right down and fell asleep. I remember the nurse coming over, putting her hand on my shoulder, and giving me a sweet look of thanks.

This was a pivotal moment for me. I thanked the Lord because He had always listened compassionately to me, and had always been merciful and comforted me, never leaving me all alone. I thought, "Wow! Here I was in the strangest, almost unreal situation, with an opportunity to spread cheer, kindness and the good news to anyone that would hear it."

"And above all these put on love, which binds everything together in perfect harmony. And let the peace of Christ rule in your hearts, to which indeed you were called in one body. And be thankful." Colossians 3:14-15

CLINGING TO HIS WORD THROUGH CANCER

This insight reminded me of when Paul and Silas were in prison. There they were, in the inner chambers of the prison, yet they were still singing and praying and praising God! They were witnesses to fellow prisoners and even to the prison guard who ultimately believed and was saved. While, I know the submarine is not a prison; I was never beaten or threatened and I knew I could go home at the end of the day. But in a similar way I believe every patient in hyperbaric felt like a prisoner to their own body. We all had this prison in common and this realization allowed me feel at ease with them. I am usually not an outgoing person, but with this change in perspective, I was ready to step out of my comfort zone and begin conversations. I was pleasantly surprised that many of the patients shared faith in our Lord and often we were an encouragement to each other. There were likely others who didn't want to hear about the good news just yet, or the opportunity to share wasn't as strong. But I felt that showing them kindness, joy, and lifting the mood was planting seeds in a small way. Little seeds of faith.

"And when they had inflicted many blows upon them, they threw them into prison, ordering the jailer to keep them safely. Having received this order, he put them into the inner prison and fastened their feet in the stocks. About midnight Paul and Silas were praying and singing hymns to God, and the prisoners were listening to them, and suddenly there was a great earthquake, so that the foundations of the prison were shaken. And immediately all the doors were opened, and everyone's bonds were unfastened. When the jailer woke and saw that the prison doors were open, he drew his sword and was about to kill himself, supposing that the prisoners had escaped. But Paul cried with a loud voice, "Do not harm

167

yourself, for we are all here." And the jailer called for lights and rushed in,

and trembling with fear he fell down before Paul and Silas. Then he

brought them out and said, "Sirs, what must I do to be saved?" And they

said, "Believe in the Lord Jesus, and you will be saved, you and your

household." And they spoke the word of the Lord to him and to all who

were in his house. And he took them the same hour of the night and

washed their wounds; and he was baptized at once, he and all his

family. Then he brought them up into his house and set food before them.

And he rejoiced along with his entire household that

he had believed in God." Acts 16: 23-34

I learned that I loved to be helpful. Each morning I would look around the submarine to see who I recognized, making small talk or picking up where our conversation had left off. But I was even more excited when there were new people. I became the unofficial greeting hostess, or "sunshine committee" for our little hyperbaric submarine. When we boarded the sub and I saw a new face I would ask if they'd ever done this before. If not, I'd explain what was about to happen. I tried introducing them to some of the others and (when I was feeling up to it) I'd even help the nurse pass out the water, chewing gum, and tissues. It wasn't a big job, but it made me feel great. I felt like I had a purpose and I was making someone's day a little better, while in turn, it made my days a lot better!

"A man who is kind benefits himself, but a cruel man hurts himself"

Proverbs 11:17

I had pneumonia at the start of my hyperbaric treatments, so by the second week of dives, my ears hurt and they hurt every day for a week! I'm not just talking a little earache; I'm talking pressure that felt like my ear drums would burst. The nurse told me that some people's eardrums actually have ruptured! Experiencing this pain, so early in my treatment, helped me learn every possible way to pop an ear. Overtime, I became known as the "expert ear popper" and that's a title I never expected to have.

As soon as a patient would start to look uncomfortable my nurses knew to walk them through with the medical advice and then they would look at me and smile. I took that as my cue to be that person's cheerleader. I'd encourage them by saying things like; "I've been there and you're doing great!" "Try yawning." "Try sipping water." I'd show them techniques and where to apply pressure and eventually their ear would pop and we had an instant bond. How strange is that?

Strange for sure, but those moments were special for me. Each morning as we drove over to the hospital I would think about who was going to be there, which nurse might be with us, and how I could make them smile. It made the entire experience much better!

During those six weeks of hyperbaric therapy, I had another surgery and several more sets of stitches. And while hyperbaric was extremely exhausting and took a lot of time every day, I can look back with thankfulness because it was a very good distraction during a very difficult healing process. I learned to spread kindness liberally, strike up conversations, and lend a helping hand even in the most unexpected of ways!

"Gracious words are like a honeycomb,

sweetness to the soul and health to the body." Proverbs 16:24

This song describes how I believed God could use me,

even in a strange place, like an indoor submarine!

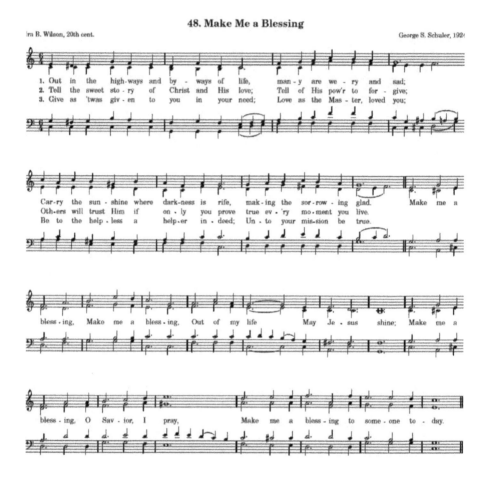

Music used with permission from "Reactor Core Hymn Repository".

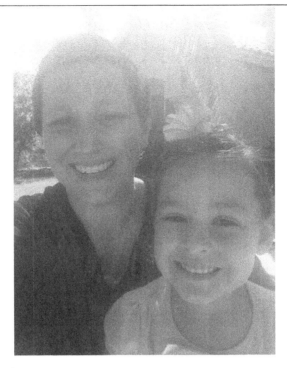

March 4th

Thankful to say, I am feeling so much better today! Thank you all for the prayers!

Sharing the words to one of my favorite hymns below, I sang it last week with a few close friends and the words are so moving, it brought me a lot of strength through this very rough post-surgery week. I hope it stays with you through the day. Following are the beautiful lyrics, to "To God Be The Glory".

My Tribute / To God Be The Glory:

"How can I say thanks; For the things You have done for me, Things so undeserved, Yet You gave to prove Your love for me.The voices of a million angels; Could not express my gratitude. All that I am and ever hope to be, I owe it all to Thee.

Chorus:

To God be the glory, To God be the glory, To God be the glory, For the things He has done. With His blood He has saved me, With His power He has raised me, To God be the glory, For the things He has done.

Verse 2

Just let me live my life, Let it be pleasing, Lord, to Thee, And if I gain any praise, Let it go to Calvary. With His blood He has saved me, With His power He has raised me, To God be the glory, For the things He has done"

March 14th: Maybe TMI for some, but I'm excited to share that this afternoon I am officially stitch free for the first time since December 30!: WooHoo! Praise God I finally feel like I'm really recovering and it feels amazing!

April 13th: Got to go to Joel's field day yesterday, Leah's field day this morning and looking forward to a field trip Friday. These are the things I've really missed the last nine months, but I'm so thankful to be doing them again. I am one grateful mama!!

"O Lord my God, I will give thanks to you forever" Psalm 30:12

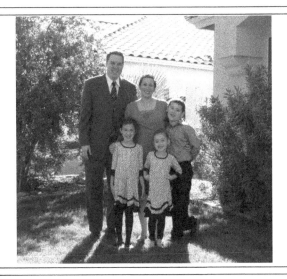

March 13th To Sunday School We Happy Go!

LAURA PENTSA

: CHAPTER 12 :
RESPECTING THE BODY GOD CREATED

I spent nearly six months of my life undergoing chemotherapy, followed by three surgeries and months of healing. I had countless appointments with the oncologists and surgeons, a handful of valuable lessons from nutritionists, and a couple training sessions with a physical trainer. Each one in their own way gave me bits of helpful information to teach me how to strengthen, heal, and respect the body God created for me.

I have taken their lessons seriously and have made many improvements to my care and nourishment, however this is an ongoing change and I am still learning this new way of life. I am not perfect, but I am getting better at developing good habits. I try to remember that slow progress is better than no progress!

Although some of the details for my diet or exercises changed throughout treatment, overall the general advice applies to everyone all the time. In fact, now working for an organization that teaches about preventive steps to lower one's risk of breast cancer, I wonder if I had respected my body and kept it healthy, would my body have been strong enough to stop the cancer when it first started? Although, I will never really know if that was the case, I do know that those same prevention techniques are what I have been taught to lower my risk of reoccurrence.

Respecting our body is very important and will make our healthy, everyday lives better. I plan to go over a general summary of what I have learned. If you want even more detail, there are tons of books dedicated specifically to nutrition, exercises, and overall wellness. Many professionals are eager to help as well.

Sleep

One of my biggest failures was not getting the sleep that my body needed. For years I stayed up way too late! Then came the kids, and there was even less sleep! In fact, I would estimate in the six years leading up to my diagnosis, I probably only slept an average of 5-6 hours on a good night, and it was rarely uninterrupted sleep. During chemotherapy my sleep cycles were sometimes complicated and hard to regulate. Napping and fatigue made a full night of sleep difficult. I knew I wanted more sleep, but had not realized how vital it was for my body. I thought sleep was just rest, but our body is actually very active while sleeping. The brain is busy locking in memories, our cells are restoring and regenerating, and our hormones are resetting. Even our moods are stabilized by having enough sleep. There are so many important functions that our bodies need to do during sleep. When we don't supply it with enough time to perform all those functions, our body's systems become unbalanced and cause a vast array of problems. As I learned about the value of sleep, I began to make it more of a priority. Some of the tips that have helped me get a longer, higher quality sleep are:

Schedule:
I've learned that I sleep better when my body is used to going to sleep and waking at approximately the same time. Before, I really didn't have a bed time, but now I have an hour window when I try to fall asleep. I usually fall asleep very quickly now. The kids and I all seem to be on the same wake schedule and we rarely even need the alarm. In fact, on Saturdays I rarely sleep more than 30 minutes longer and wake up feeling very well rested, which is a great indicator that I am getting a good amount of sleep all week long.

Darken the room:

I was taught that sleeping in a dark room promotes a healthy level of melatonin. Melatonin is a hormone produced by a gland in the brain while you sleep. This hormone does a lot of work during the night to set your sleep cycle. I also found using a very small dose of supplemental melatonin was extremely helpful at times. I found melt-away tablets and I just bite off the small amount that I need for a good night sleep. Since I am quite sensitive, I like that I could adjust the dose for specifically what my body needed and take just enough to doze off without feeling overly drowsy the next day.

Start winding down:

At least an hour before sleeping I try to completely relax. No more chores, no more emails, no more projects. I just sit or lay down and rest.

Get comfy:

The body temperature naturally drops down during the night, so having a warm blanket keeps me in a deep sleep, and I'm not wrestling around to get warm. In the summer when it's really hot, I've learned that it is well worth the cost to lower the thermostat down an extra couple degrees so that I'm comfortable. I found that after my mastectomy I had to change my sleep habits and could no longer sleep on my stomach. Sleeping on my side with a body pillow has become my new normal.

Food

I got more advice about what I should eat and what I should not eat from professionals, family, friends, acquaintances, and yes, even strangers. It seemed like the second people found out I had cancer, everyone wanted to tell me how their great aunt's best friend's cousin didn't need chemo because she had a rare organic green plant extract collected by nuns, hand-pressed and delivered via angels to her bedside... OK, obviously I am exaggerating, but I heard many over-the-top recommendations by very well-meaning people. They were people who wanted to help, but had no idea how overwhelming and exhausting all of this information actually was. If I stopped eating everything that someone had told me could possibly cause or make the cancer worse, I'd probably be left with 2 or 3 raw vegetables to choose from. If I started taking every supplement that someone told me I had to try, I'd have been taking pills by the handful. All of this to say there is a lot of information out there about food and nutrition. I am only going to touch on the aspects that all of my medical team seemed to be in agreement on.

The lifestyle changes I had to implement surround a low fat, high fiber, low sugar plan. Sounds fun right? It takes effort, thought, and planning to live this way. I am still not where I want to be with my diet, but I am leaps and bounds from where I started. I actually thought I ate pretty well before I had cancer. I like fruits and vegetables, I like to cook, and I've learned how to read a nutrition label pretty well. Having polycystic ovarian syndrome my entire adult life, I've always struggled with the weight around my midsection and have been on many diets and had to watch what I eat. Even so, now looking back, I still was not even close to this new way of living. I've been making changes to nourish and respect my body.

Women have been telling their children for generations, "Eat your vegetables" and it is time we take our own advice! This is probably the most important piece of advice a person can get when it comes to nutrition, and it seems so obvious that it is easy to ignore. Our bodies need around 5-6 servings of vegetables per day! Very few Americans actually fill their bodies with this amount of good-high fiber, low calorie, vitamin-packed nutrition. The bulk of our food throughout the day should really be vegetables. Then comes fruit at about 3-4 servings per day. I personally find that much easier and more enjoyable, but both are critical! Many people are walking around "full" yet completely malnourished! We require dozens of minerals and vitamins, plus amino and fatty acids for our body to work properly and function at full capacity. To meet that need, we need a large array of vegetables and fruit. My nutritionist spent time teaching me about the phytochemicals that fresh produce supply to our bodies. Think of these as the edible rainbow. Phytochemicals fuel the immune system and neutralize cancer-causing substances. They support our overall health by strengthening our immune system and blood vessels and by fighting tumors. Now I brighten up my plate. I eat a lot of green, but I also include so many other bright beautiful fruits and vegetables. Some people really hate their vegetables and I would encourage them to keep trying, but some other ways to get your servings in quickly are organic juices (cold pressed are best), smoothies, or even "green" powder mixes. These are all good too, but really nothing is as filling or as nutritious and high in fiber as the raw natural produce. Something that should be remembered is that during chemotherapy, don't eat too many antioxidants because they do such a good job at protecting cells that it may prevent the chemotherapy from damaging the cancer cells, which is the goal! A great way to avoid this problem is to eat a vast variety of fruits and vegetables. Don't limit yourself to just one or two types. Variety will help provide lots of great nutrition, but not overload you in one area! When chemotherapy is complete then you can ramp up the antioxidants for overall healing! However, variety is still important!

The next biggest category is whole grains. The more complex and less processed the better. Four servings is a healthy goal. Grains are high in fiber, give us energy, and keep us full and satisfied. I avoid white or highly processed breads and flours as they are broken down completely differently in our bodies and don't supply any of the same benefits. Good whole grain options are whole wheat, oats, quinoa, farro, buckwheat, bulgur, barley, brown rice, whole couscous and chia. These are usually high in fiber and nutrition.

I've learned to decrease the portions of all other food categories. The amount of meat I eat, six oz per day, is a healthy target. I now opt for lower fat options including skinless chicken and turkey, lean pork tenderloin, nitrate-free lunchmeat, lean beef or 90-96% lean ground beef, and most varieties of seafood.

Grilling is a wonderful option because it really decreases the amount of fat, but you need to use a marinade or heavy dry rub. My nutritionist said that by coating the meat it dramatically decreases the carcinogens. I avoid sugary marinades as they can have the same or worse chemical reaction that the meat has. Instead, I use a thin vinegar or olive oil based marinade with herbs and spices. I enjoy using Italian dressings,
citrus herb blends, and chimichurri sauce as marinades. I've also learned to avoid flare ups and cut off charred portions, because they contain more carcinogens.

I also decreased the amount of cheese I eat and look for lower fat options. I use an egg substitute frequently since that is also lower in fat grams than regular eggs. I try to limit low-fat milk and yogurt to two servings per day.

I have replaced white sugar and it is rarely used in our home. We rely on pure maple syrup and honey as our sweeteners. And occasionally we use other more natural, low-calorie sweeteners like stevia, erythritol and xylitol, pretty much in that order. I have had to experiment with baking and how these sugars affect the recipes, but it can be done.

When I am somewhere and sweets are out, I do allow myself a little bit. I have learned that if I don't indulge a little bit then I just keep obsessing about it until I really lose control. I've learned to aim for healthy choices at least 80% of the time and give myself a break the other 20%. A good health advocate and friend gave me that little tip and it makes living this way much less stressful. Find the percentage that is right for you, and maybe you can even follow the plan 90%. Just do your best.

Lastly, fats! This one sneaks its way into so many things. I aim to have less than three servings per day, and hope to make good choices using monounsaturated fats rather than other less-desirable fats. These healthy fats include avocado, peanut butter, oils, nuts, olives, and pesto sauce. Limiting these to three per day is still very difficult for me. I try to avoid the unhealthy polyunsaturated fats like mayonnaise and many salad dressings or the saturated fats like bacon, butter, and cream cheese. Other fats that I completely avoid are trans fats or partially hydrogenate fat products. I had to really learn and practice reading every nutrition label. With practice, this too is getting easier.

♡♡♡

When I was sick and people wanted to help with meals, I was concerned because the typical casseroles are not full of vegetables and are often high in fat. Thankfully, my Aunt Corinne (my support team organizer) sent out my food requests to anyone who volunteered to help. I mostly preferred grocery drop-offs. A couple bags of cleaned and prepared fresh produce, with a bag of whole wheat bread, nitrate-free lunch meat, and 1% milk for our family was dropped off twice per week. That worked really well. My husband or mom often grilled us dinner and the fresh vegetables and fruit were our sides. The sandwiches made for easy lunches and the milk and fruit for easy breakfasts. With everything prepped, I could usually handle plating up the meals and getting everyone fed. When even this was too difficult, post-surgery, we asked for cooked meals. Aunt Corinne sent out a list of our favorite meal choices and many people were happy to help. Another helpful option for people that wanted to provide a meal but didn't have the ability or time to cook, was a list of what our family orders from our favorite take out restaurants. Only a couple people used those suggestions and it was helpful and a nice change of pace. I will include our food lists that we sent out to our helpers. I am thankful that I asked for what specifically worked for our family and would recommend others to request what is best for them too.

Meal Sign up for the Pentsa Family

During the month of January we would like to provide a delivery of fresh fruits and vegetables to Dave on each Sunday and two prepared meals delivered to their home, each Tuesday & Friday around **5:00**.

If you would like to provide a meal – please see the below menu suggestions. There is also an attached sheet for Take-Out options. Please indicate on the sign-up sheet what meal you will be providing so that we don't give them too much of the same thing all at once.

☐ Grilled Meat (Chicken, Beef or Pork) with brown rice, asparagus & a salad

☐ Baked Chicken with noodles, cooked carrots & salad

☐ Spaghetti & Meatballs or Meat-Sauce with green beans & Caesar salad

☐ Soft Tacos: wheat tortillas with ground beef; lettuce, tomato, shredded cheese with chips, salsa & sour cream. Salad; lettuce with Pico de Gallo

☐ Lasagna, side of sliced cucumbers and salad

☐ Pot Roast cooked with lots of carrots, celery, onions, potatoes

☐ Chicken Broccoli Divan over brown rice with salad

If you would like to provide the fresh fruits and vegetables, there is also an attached list of preferred foods.

Please use DISPOSABLE PANS

Sunday – Jan. 3rd   Fresh Fruit & Veggies _____

Tuesday – Jan. 5th   Meal: _____

Friday – Jan. 8th   Meal: _____

If you would like to provide a dessert, here are some family favorites: Popsicles; Chocolate Pudding; Fruit Salad; Strawberry Shortcake; Yogurt Parfaits; Chocolate covered fruit

If you would like to purchase a meal and deliver it to their home, here are some family favorites:

Boston Market: $32.45
Rotisserie Chicken Family Meal for 4: 1 ¼ chicken
4 large sides: Sweet Potatoes, Creamed Spinach, Green Beans, Macaroni & Cheese; 4 Cornbread

Chipotle: $25.75 :Qt. 1 : Steak Burrito with brown rice, pinto beans, fresh tomato salsa, sour cream, cheese, and lettuce Qty. 1: Barbacoa Burrito Bowl with brown rice, black beans, roasted chilli-corn salsa, sour cream, cheese, lettuce Qty. 3: Steak Taco in soft flour tortilla, Fresh tomato salsa, sour cream, cheese and Lettuce. Qty. 1: Chips and Guacamole

Vitamins

Even eating well, sometimes our bodies still need help getting all of the necessary minerals and vitamins. Vitamin D seems to be a very common problem in cancer patients. Vitamin D helps bodies absorb other important minerals including calcium and phosphorous for strong bones, it keeps the immune system going, and helps to fight off certain diseases. Going outside and getting some sunshine is an easy, natural way to get Vitamin D. Unfortunately even living in sunny Arizona, my body is still very deficient, so I need to take a supplement. I prefer to take a liquid vitamin D or the pill form with coconut oil to aid in absorption. I have had blood tests that taught me other beneficial supplements and I take a general daily vitamin. Helping my body get the nutrients it was lacking is one easy thing I can do for my health.

Stay Hydrated

I learned to drink water all throughout the day. On average most people should be drinking eight 8oz glasses of water per day. I have found that I love drinking from a huge 32oz mason jar and that way if I refill once and drink it all then I know I've done well and had enough water for the day. I don't always care for the taste of water, but I've found ways to make water more appealing. Some of my favorites are: citrus fruit, herbs, teas, flavor mixes, etc... There are lot of ways to flavor water without adding sugar.

Exercise

"One step at a time." "You can do this!" "Set a goal and hit it." "Just 5 more minutes." "Keep going!" "I am getting stronger!" These are the motivational mantras I say to myself all the time. I have never loved to exercise, but I am learning to love the feeling of accomplishment. When I had cancer, I often heard about the benefits of staying active and exercise, but some days, it really wasn't possible to do much. I think it is important to make yourself get up, and get moving as much as you can. My caring sister-in-law Jenn came to help when I was almost done with chemo and my body was very weak. I had asked her to go for a walk with me

> *Just keep trying!*

because I was so bored of being inside. That day we walked along about 5 houses when my legs started to tremble and I started to feel a bit dizzy. With her at my side, we did get back home and I napped for most of the afternoon. Compared to where I am now, fully healed and healthy, I could run past those 5 houses and back home and only be slightly winded. But, on that day, this was as far as I could safely push myself. I think that is the key - to keep pushing, keep trying, but also know your limits. After treatment was over, my oncologist recommended that I aim to exercise 40 minutes, 5 days a week. I am still not there yet, but I am getting closer. I am getting stronger and eventually I know I will be capable of that. It's been a year and sometimes I do feel like a failure that I haven't met that goal, but then I have to remind myself of how far I've really come. A year ago, I was just getting over surgery, still stitched up and still incredibly weak. Now, 1 year later, I walk the kids to the park and back and it is actually very easy.

Just keep trying! Our bodies need us to do this for so many reasons, but to me this is just another important way of showing respect to the body I am so blessed to have.

Reduce Chemicals

I used to love to trying new shampoos, lotions, and cleaning supplies. I can remember going down the hygiene aisle at the grocery store when my last bottle had emptied and loving to pick out the next new bottle. Maybe I'm weird that I loved this so much, but looking at all the pretty bottles and opening the lid to puff up what the scent smelled like was fun for me. I even thought I was being pretty health-minded when

I'd pick out one that said something like "natural" or "organic" on the packaging. Naively, I thought living in an advanced country, that anything I picked would be relatively safe. Unfortunately, I was wrong. Many cosmetic, hygienic and cleaning products contain cancer-causing ingredients. It is left to the consumer to read the label and decode the ingredients. I learned how to read a nutrition label, but I'd have to become a chemist to know what I'm reading when I look at the back of a cosmetic label. Here are a couple good tips that have helped me to know what is safe:

First, the shorter and more readable the ingredient list, the safer the product is likely to be. I also learned to count the commas. Many times a common name is listed, then followed by the scientific name and it starts to become really confusing. But if you count the commas, you'll more easily figure out how many ingredients are actually inside. When I am choosing a lotion and the label shows 35 ingredients, I look for a better choice and switch to one that lists only 12. Even better, I've learned that there are often natural remedies that work just as well. For a good moisturizer, I only need one ingredient! I like coconut oil or Shea butter.

Second, I try to skip things that use the generic term "Fragrance". Often they do not say what it is because the list would be far too long, it is made with synthetic chemicals or possibly they might not want you to know what is really in there. Many things labeled "Fragrance" do contain carcinogens. Instead I try looking for products that actually list real floral, herbal scents or essential oils.

Product research

My boss, Holly, introduced me to the Environmental Working Group at EWG.org. It is a wealth of information regarding the toxicity of products and can help you find similar safer products. It is a wonderful tool for looking up health grades for these products. EWG's "Skindeep" website catalogs cosmetic products to find out their overall rating, and I look one step further at the cancer concern. If it is moderate to high for cancer concern then it is not something I want in my home.

The same concept is also available for cleaning supplies in "EWG's Guide to Healthy Cleaning" and food with "EWG's Healthy Living". Now when I need to replace a product I look up a superior, safer choice. I am more educated and am happy knowing our home has fewer toxins.

Avoid pesticides

This is a hard one for my household. We live in the desert and our backyard is right against a wash (what we call a dry creek bed). It is a beautiful desert landscape, but it comes with critters, and my least favorite: scorpions! Now for me, I have to weigh the decision of watching my footsteps for scorpions or having pesticides out along the edge of our property. I do choose pesticides.

However, this doesn't mean I welcome pesticides inside our home, our refrigerator or worst of all, our bodies. While it cannot be completely avoided, I do try to shop organic when possible. This includes skincare because the skin is the body's largest organ. I also try to buy organic when it comes to the "Dirty Dozen". This includes strawberries, apples, nectarines, peaches, celery, grapes, cherries, spinach, tomatoes, bell peppers, cherry tomatoes, cucumbers, hot peppers and kale. These produce items have the most residual pesticides, so buying organic is a good choice. If organic is too costly or not available, I am sure to wash the fruit very well with a fruit and vegetable spray wash or rinse with vinegar (I hate the smell of vinegar so I love my fruit wash!)

Limit plastics

It seems like almost everything now comes wrapped in plastic. Even healthy snacks are wrapped in plastic! While I have not been able to completely avoid them, I try to control plastics where I can. I have been slowly switching our kitchen to a plastic-free zone. In particular, plastics labeled with the recycle code 3 or 7 are far from healthy, so I try to keep those out of our home and especially away from our food. The type of plastic is not always clearly indicated, so I have been attempting to slowly replace our kitchen plastics with stainless steel or glass. I wish I'd started my kitchen out that way. Stainless steel and glass are easier to clean, they don't stain, and they don't melt. Overall I'm really happy with this change.

Habits

Smoking and alcohol habit changes are difficult to make. Thankfully, I never started these habits. But I am sure for many this would not be easy. To state it simply, please stop smoking! Professionals have said this over and over, yet I know it still happens. Find help and quit! Secondly, make alcohol a special treat. If you choose to drink alcoholic beverages, limit your weekly consumption to three servings per week. One serving equals five oz of wine or 12 oz of beer, or one and a half oz of distilled alcohol.

Ask your medical team for specific portion sizes and recommendations customized to fit your needs. They can answer questions directly or refer you to an expert for help.

This summary of caring for the body was still quite a lot of information, but it really does make a huge difference to health and healing. While I was sick, I wanted my body to have every advantage at fighting and keeping strong. Once I was well, I wanted it to stay that way! I hope my experiences and personal learning curve can be an advantage to others and help form good habits. God has miraculously formed our bodies and we are given the precious responsibility of caring for them.

"Be strong, and let your heart take courage,

all you who wait for the LORD!" Psalm 31:24

LAURA PENTSA

⦂ CHAPTER 13 ⦂
CELEBRATE!

I doubt I'm alone in loving a beautiful celebration! Not everyone loves weddings and baby showers the way I do, but I definitely look forward to every occasion to celebrate. When I was sick and going through treatment, I recall friends saying things like, "Just think, one day this will all be done and we will have so much to look back on and be thankful for". This planted a tiny idea that proved to be a huge inspiration and a wonderful goal to focus on. I decided that if, at the end of treatment I was well enough, that I would host a huge celebration.

I would think about the celebration when my treatment or recovery caused me to miss a special event, or when going to the doctor and I was wanting to be anywhere else. I often thought: "Well, I might have to miss out on this, but I'll make sure to invite them to my celebration and we will all be together".

I recall a breast cancer survivor saying that when she had to miss out on an event because of treatment, each time she would put a bead in a jar. When she went into remission at the end of treatment , she then used those same beads to make a necklace. Each time she got the opportunity to go out and enjoy a children's program, a party, or a date with her husband, she would put one of those beads on her necklace. Soon she ran out, but with each new bead she bought she continued to recognize her blessings. She would pause and give thanks that the treatment had worked and now she could have many more of those events and special moments!

While I never personally collected beads or made a necklace, that image stayed with me and I'd think that while I may be missing out on something today, I will have my celebration and many more after that. Keeping this positive goal ahead of me really helped get me through some lonely days. I am so incredibly thankful that one year later, I know I have an entire necklace-worth of "invisible" beads, many precious moments when I paused to be grateful.

If I couldn't sleep at night then I would go on Pinterest.com, and look at party ideas. (No, this was not one of my tips for a good quality night sleep, but perhaps when all else fails... then comes Pinterest!?!) Some nights, when I couldn't fall asleep, I'd look up decorations, recipes, party favors, etc. I'd have to throw a dozen parties to use all of the great ideas that I'd "pinned." I smiled, fantasizing over the big celebration day. Honestly, I spent SO much more time thinking about this party than I even did planning our wedding!

I got a pink notebook to fill with ideas. I had the recipes, layout design, pictures, and guests list. It was over the top, but it was very good for me. I'd browse through beautiful pictures, thinking about a positive outcome and I'd fall asleep very happy. I believe those positive thoughts helped when I could have encountered some very dark, troubling evenings. This party brought me happiness months before the real planning could really begin.

Ironically, when the actual day of the party arrived, my plans all flew out the window. Living in Phoenix, I planned that the party would be held in my beautiful backyard. When I say planned, it was down to the last detail! However, as we set up the decor that day, the dark clouds came and went, came and went, and finally came and stayed. I must admit, after all of the planning and preparation, I shed quite a few tears at the thought of throwing out those perfect plans and going to a much less liked, much less planned, "Plan B"! We quickly decided to have the bulk of the party inside with only overflow seating outside. Brian, my brother-in-law, saved the day with a quick last-minute call for a rental canopy that we definitely ended up needing! While the rain poured, my sweet sister-in-law Jenn, pointed out a quote I had printed and put into a pink frame that I'd painted weeks before, planning to use as a decoration at the party. The quote was,

"Life isn't about waiting for the storms to pass...
it's about learning to dance in the rain." -Unknown

I am so glad she reminded me of this quote! It was perfect and completely snapped me out of my resistance to change plans. Now looking back, even knowing that many of the plans would go unused, I wouldn't change it. All of the planning gave me so much happiness, anticipation, and excitement. The evening turned out perfect, even through the storm. The flowers my mom affectionately arranged in hand-decoupaged mason jars were still stunning! The Mexican meal that Dave's mom oversaw was completely delicious! The perfect pink baked goods our church ladies lovingly made were still decedent! The honey jars Annette and Melanie helped tenderly wrap with a favorite verse were just right! The cotton candy maker and canopy Brian provided kept the backyard going, even in the rain! All of the many other details my sweet-sister-in-laws Jenn and Adrienne worked at were lovely, and helped pull it all together! I had wanted to do all of this by myself as a gift to all of them for their loving support through the year. But instead, just like they had before, so many gathered round, to help me again. They served and supported us as they had over and over throughout the year. The day of the celebration, their love for me and my family was brightly shining through the rain.

In the months leading up to the party, my purpose for the celebration began to change. At first it was: "Let's throw a party that cancer is over!" To: "Let's throw a party that teaches breast cancer awareness". To finally "Let's throw a party to end this chapter with thankfulness for all of the people who helped us!" This last one felt right and it became even more inspiring to me.

I knew I couldn't possibly send a gift to every person who provided groceries, a meal, a service, or who drove me somewhere, babysat, or helped financially. I found it difficult to even stay on top of Thank You notes during certain points of treatment (sorry to any who never received one!). When people would help or show support, I wanted to thank them at my celebration. I wanted to host the party as a giant thank you gift; a tribute to everyone who helped bring my family through this. I am so thankful because I truly believe everyone there understood my intent and walked away feeling our gratitude and sincere appreciation. It was an emotional event, in the best possible way. On the night of the celebration, before a champagne toast, I spoke these few words to our many honored guests:

"Everyone, thank you so much for coming here tonight to celebrate with us! I am not much for public speaking, but this year I learned I can do some pretty scary things, so I am going to try! After all, you are all my friends.

There are so many reasons to be celebrating tonight. I celebrate the fact that I am well enough to do something like this, that I am able to go for walks and help at the school and just be a normal mom again! I celebrate every morning that I wake up and get to teach my kids a little bit more! And even though my health alone is a wonderful reason to celebrate it is not really the reason I wanted to throw this party.

I really wanted to celebrate tonight as a tribute to all the support I had, to the many who have made a really ugly illness into something bright and beautiful. I wanted to cook you all dinner and provide you a night of joy as a thank you gift for the many ways you have blessed me and my family.

A tribute to:

A God who is so BIG & SO mighty, yet He loves even me! And He loves you too!

A Savior who gives me HOPE! Not hope for just a cure, but eternal HOPE!

A Spirit who comforts even when pain & exhaustion take their physical toll.

My family who gave over & over their continuous time, energy, & support!

My friends far & near who prayed on our behalf & encouraged us everyday!

My church family who stepped in to help wherever & whenever! Caring for us in every possible way!

The medical team who treated me with knowledge, compassion, and confidence!

The kids' teachers who taught & cared for them so I didn't have to worry while I napped!

The many that have "done Cancer before" and taught me how to do this with joy and a smile!

To ALL of you... Thank you!!!! Every single way you've

shown your care and love is special and means so much
to us!"

    I guess for me, planning the celebration was a blessing in and of itself, and the actual event was a moment in my life which I'll never ever forget! It really was the perfect way for me to close the chapter of daily treatment and sickness, thank everyone who helped along the way, and then wake up the next morning ready to step into the next chapter of life!

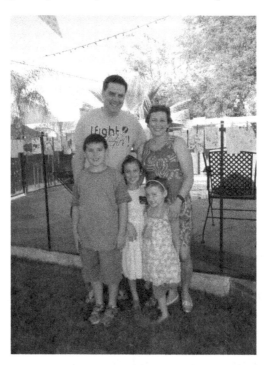

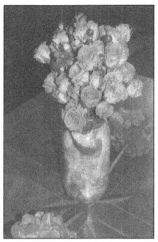 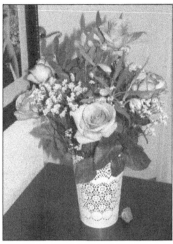

My mom arranged dozens of these!
They were all over the house and yard!

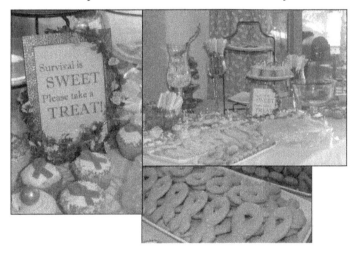

My Aunt Marta made dozens of beautiful, pink
baked goods and enlisted the help of our loving
church friends who were among our biggest
supporters throughout the year!

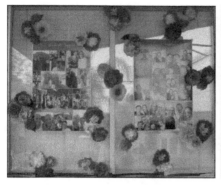
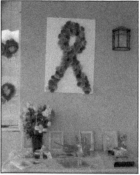

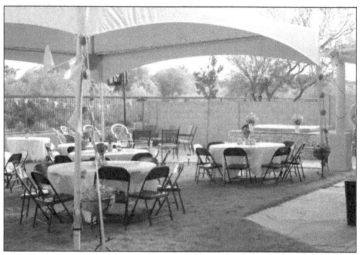

The backyard, all decorated and ready,
come rain or shine!

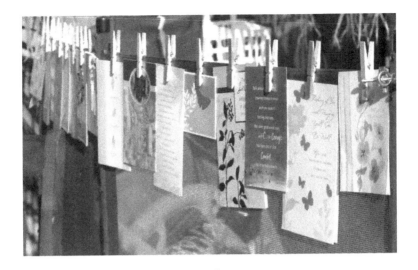

My favorite part of the decorations were the cards. The cards lined our entire pool fence! The party was surrounded with the encouragment and well-wishes people had sent me through the year! I loved my cards!

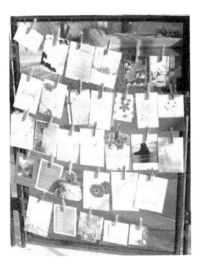

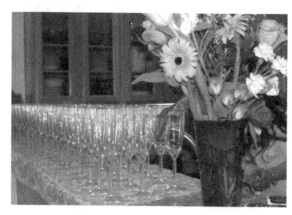

My tribute of
thanks followed
by a champagne
toast

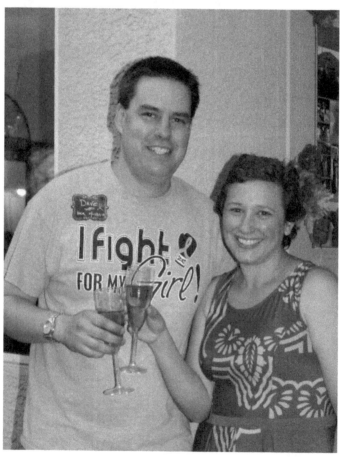

"Therefore, since we have been justified by faith, we have peace with God through our Lord Jesus Christ. Through him we have also obtained access by faith into this grace in which we stand, and we rejoice in hope of the glory of God. Not only that, but we rejoice in our sufferings, knowing that suffering produces endurance, and endurance produces character, and character produces hope, and hope does not put us to shame, because God's love has been poured into our hearts through the Holy Spirit who has been given to us"

Romans 8:24-25

LAURA PENTSA

: CHAPTER 14 :
BRINGING LESSONS INTO SURVIVORSHIP

After the celebration party, I neatly closed the chapter of my life entitled 'cancer'. I was so excited for it to be completely finished and to move forward into the next chapter of survivorship!

Thankfully today, I can report that I'm healthy, strong, and filled with gratitude. My family is able to play games, be active, travel and stay busy, all with me right beside them! I am able to participate at church, volunteer at the kids' school, and am even back to work. My life is now very busy with so many good things. This was what I expected survivorship to continually look like. While it does most of the time, there are still the physical reminders cancer has left behind. I needed to carry the lessons from Queen Esther, King David, and Apostle Paul with me into this new chapter of life. I needed to stay rooted in God's love and His Holy Word because there are still some hard moments in survivorship. And, this new chapter quickly proved that life is rarely neat or tidy. I am still learning what life after cancer really looks like.

For example within the same week of my party I was already back at my oncology surgeon's office in a near-panic. My right breast (the trouble-maker) was acting up again. I woke up one morning and noticed a huge lump, unlike the one I felt before, right there on the surface - ugly and undeniable. By the time I got to the doctor's office it had actually opened, oozed, and left a strange flap of skin behind, kind of like a blister.

"What is this?!?!" "Did the cancer come back?!?!" I was desperate for an immediate answer. Thankfully, my doctor was certain it was not cancer and she was confident that it was only an abscess or boil. When my skin started to heal, the tiny hair follicles became inflamed and infected. No big deal! I am learning that my recovery and survivorship is full of these "no big deal" moments, that for a short time feel like an extremely big deal!

My year since treatment has had plenty of these jaw-dropping, heart-stopping moments. All of the sudden a fear of reoccurrence can slap me silly! Almost every day someone will ask, "Laura how are you doing now?" Usually my response is; "I am thankful to be doing very well, getting better and stronger all the time." This really is my new normal, thankfully so. But I never seem to know just what curveball my body will throw at me, or which test result might signal red flags. I've learned that my body is still recovering so sometimes these things just pop up.

I've also learned that when I freak out, that it is okay. This is a perfectly normal, human response. Our bodies are designed to be protective. I am perfectly normal to feel this way and to even struggle with paranoia from time to time. "Is that pain normal?" "Did my skin always look that way?" "Does this feel different than it did yesterday?" To an outsider who never heard the words: "You have cancer", these questions probably do sound completely paranoid and obsessive. But to someone who has lived through cancer as their own reality, these questions not only make sense but are a part of responsible observations.

> *Tip: Learn to track and document body changes that concern you. I even mark these on my calendar, if the problem is still persisting one week later, I make an appointment with my doctor.*

The vivid memory of finding my cancerous lump in the shower one perfectly normal day, and thinking that it was nothing, can sometimes terrify me. I had almost ignored that lump. I almost convinced myself not to bother with an appointment. I almost made a grave mistake. I don't want to gloss over anything now.

So where does all of this lead me? Am I a total mess? Am I constantly living in fear? NO WAY! When these surprises happen, I may go into momentary shock and panic, but then I act. I call my doctor and ask a question, or I take a measurement and a picture to track physical changes over the next couple days, or I make an appointment to have a professional decide what's next.

Sure, it's stressful. And at times I worry that I may look like a hypochondriac. But who cares? I'd rather know my own body and catch something early on than wait while my "stage" could be changing. Knowing that my doctors will see me, run tests, and continue checking up on me takes the stress away from the rest of my normal and mostly-great days. My advice would be to act and find out quickly, so you can move on to the good stuff! While waiting on a symptom to subside or an appointment to arrive, I'd aim to think on the good things and not let these physical symptoms take up too much of my thoughts. Worry does not change anything for the better. These are the times to again remember to turn to the Lord in prayer, song, and praise.

"Blessed is the man who remains steadfast under trial,

for when he has stood the test he will receive the crown of life,

which God has promised to those who love him." James 1:12

Coming to love my new normal has also taken a great deal of adjusting. Everyone heals in their own way and at a different pace. Most would agree that we all want to be healed yesterday. However, being patient on healing can be really hard. Some side effects lingered on much longer than I wanted. I can remember just wanting my eyelashes to be long again. I remember when they first started to "sprout" and I was SO excited. I looked in the mirror every day just hoping they'd magically grow overnight and be long, full and beautiful. After one year, they are still very short! My eyelashes grow really slowly, but I am really thankful to have them back.

Waiting for my hair to grow has also been a lesson in patience, too. Going from bald, to fuzz, to pixie, to curly, to awkward has been a unique experience. There were days I've been frustrated waiting for it to grow, wanting it to look different. On those days I could easily turn my negative attitude around. I just looked at one of the bald pictures I had from chemotherapy. Suddenly, I remembered how thankful I was to have my hair back, even if it still wasn't the full length I once had. "Ah-ha!...Look at all my beautiful hair!" Now, I try to remind myself of the many blessings good health has restored and to be mindful not to take them for granted.

"... we rejoice in our sufferings, knowing that suffering produces endurance,

and endurance produces character, and character produces hope, and

hope does not put us to shame, because God's love has been poured into

our hearts through the Holy Spirit who has been given to us." Romans 5:3-5

There are also the new normals that are more difficult to get used to. For one, the fatigue that hasn't completely gone away. It's much better, but I am still hit with fatigue unlike any I experienced before cancer. I'm learning to not expect myself to function at the same level as two years ago, and I am learning to live within my limits.

Spontaneous neuropathy seems to strike when I get cold or too tired. I don't know if I'll ever get used to the numbness or worse (to me) - the stingy, tingling sensation in my fingers and toes. I still feel embarrassed at how often I drop things or lose my grip. It is my new normal, but because it comes and goes, I never really get used to it.

I now need to wear eyeglasses because hyperbaric pressure changed the shape of my eye, a change that continually reminds me of all I've been through.

Another lasting side effect that I hope will someday disappear is the sudden electric shock that suddenly zaps through my breasts. I've come to understand that this is just nerve damage, but it's never expected and is always a bit alarming.

And the awful chemo brain! The chemotherapy medications can cause cellular and nerve damage, even effecting the thought process. The memory lapses, getting my words all mixed up, or needing a calculator for simple arithmetic is the new normal. My memory wasn't great before, but I would love to go back to that.

My new calendar is still filled with regularly scheduled doctors appointments. Check ups every three months with three different doctors, blood work, and follow up scans constantly rotating which means that I am still in the doctors office a lot. As I pass this one year anniversary, some of the appointments will start to extend out to six months, and that sounds much better to me.

"For those who live according to the flesh set their minds on the things of the flesh, but those who live according to the Spirit set their minds on the things of the Spirit. For to set the mind on the flesh is death, but to set the mind on the Spirit is life and peace." Romans 8:5-6

There are many other little changes that I have begun to accept as a part of my new normal, but there is one change that I wonder if I will ever be able to look past. My mastectomy scars. Walking out of my shower, my bathroom might as well be a circus fun house. We have two oval mirrors that reflect right at the shower doors, a large full-length mirror to the left, and a small medicine cabinet mirror to the right. When I get dressed outside of our shower, I can't help but see my scars from every angle. It used to be upsetting to me, and while I am now somewhat numb to it, my eye goes straight to the scars. I don't even see the rest of me, I just see those lines, the leftover symbols of everything I went through. My stretch marks speak reminders of my children, but those mastectomy scars scream reminders of surgery, stitches (and stitches and stitches), and hyperbaric. Whether they feel like it or not, these are a part of my new normal.

♡♡♡

This new normal might sound horrible, but please don't misunderstand - not all of these physical concerns happen every day, and most are simply a momentary reminder of what I've been through. I could have skipped over writing about this part of survivorship, but I want this book to be honest and the complete truth. There are the parts of survivorship that are hard, but that is a very small price to pay for all of the many good things that have also become even bigger parts of my new normal!

My survivorship is not only full of good health, and a body that can do almost anything I'd ever want, but more importantly, my survivorship is full of the precious life lessons that I learned rapidly during treatment. These are lessons that I'd have otherwise needed years to learn. I feel much older and wiser than I did when I was diagnosed and I am incredibly grateful for my growth. Gaining so much insight during cancer truly taught me how little I actually know. If I could learn this much this quickly, then the lessons and answers of this world are unlimited.

Thankfully, I know The One, who holds every answer. I know the Lord who is omniscient. I trust Him to know everything, and don't need to worry that I don't. I am thankful that He has taught me so much, and am thankful that I am still learning!

"He determines the number of the stars; He gives to all of them their names.

Great is our Lord, and abundant in power; His understanding

is beyond measure." Psalm 147: 4-5

♡♡♡

Lessons Learned

I learned that my voice is worth something. I am not perfect by any means and don't claim to have all the answers, but the Lord has been teaching me lessons! I knew these lessons were a gift that I should not selfishly keep to myself. I wanted to share what He had lovingly taught me through this difficult experience. Though I never had much confidence speaking publicly, the Lord had shown me other ways to share these lessons. Through written word, being an example, and in my everyday conversations I can pass these lessons on to others. This lesson gave me more courage to not be silent, and to speak up or write a message of value or encouragement.

Keeping these lessons to myself would be squandering the new opportunities that the Lord has blessed me with. I do not want any to be wasted. It may have seemed emotionally easier to go through this same diagnosis and treatment without opening up to everyone, or shoving down the emotions, keeping it all secret or feeling bad for myself. I'm thankful for the lessons from Queen Esther that inspired me to be open. Everyone's support proved to be a blessing to me and I pray that my experience has blessed others.

I learned to see opportunity in asking what the Lord could make out of such a unique and trying time. I prayed that God would use this awful diagnosis for His own glory and for something good and believe in many ways He did and He is still being glorified through it.

Life is full of struggles. I urge you to not waste opportunities, find ways to draw close to the Lord through them, learn from them and use these lessons to help others.

"And above all these put on love, which binds everything together in perfect harmony. And let the peace of Christ rule in your hearts, to which indeed you were called in one body. And be thankful." Colossians 3:14-15

I now appreciate my body and am amazed at the miraculous creation we are. God designed us in an intricate way, down to our DNA. Yet, each of us were created with a custom body, mind and spirit. This is completely mind boggling. Having spent a little time learning about cancer and nutrition, I am in awe of what He has created. Our bodies are magnificent masterpieces and I am honored and privileged to have been given one to care for.

I learned to consider what I eat and my perspective on nutrition has completely changed. In the past, I dieted to lose weight. Now I care more about fueling my body, making sure to provide the essential nutrients that help it function and feel better. I like the feeling of accomplishment and knowing I've made a healthier choice. I learned to identify progress by what I am capable of doing and how long or how fast I can go, rather than solely by weight loss. This new perspective feels great and empowering. I am thankful for this new perspective. Good health is an exceptionally special gift. A well-functioning body is precious and I was foolish not to treat it better before facing cancer.

"I can do all things through him who strengthens me." Philippians 4:13

I learned that I can choose to look at things from a positive perspective. Self-control involves not just my physical body, but also my mind and spirit. I can think on good things!

Even small inspirations can be of huge importance to attitude and perspective. Like with my greeting cards, which brought me so much comfort and cheer. I worked for a greeting card company for seven years, yet never knew just how important they could actually be. Cards may seem insignificant, but to me they were wonderful. Filled with well wishes and scripture, each card was healing emotionally, spiritually, and at times physically as they helped change my focus and perspective. I loved those cards and it was like being spoon-fed scripture one verse at-a-time and being hugged by someone from far away.

"...giving thanks always and for everything to God the Father

in the name of our Lord Jesus Christ," Ephesians 5:20

I learned that I can ALWAYS find something to be thankful for. Even in unpleasant physical reminders of what cancer has done to my body, I can be reminded to be grateful. Grateful that those are only scars of my past, that today my health is restored, that I have energy and the desire to fully take life in.

There are also the effortless reminders of how much I have to be thankful for. Watching our incredibly beautiful kids grow and flourish, listening to them and knowing that they are also wise beyond their years because of this time of trial. They have grown in their own faith in God. They appreciate our family and find joy in simple pleasures. They are building character and have been able to witness us cling to God's Holy Word in times of trial. They have learned to really pray and talk to the Lord. The children are still young, and this is all just the start of their growth, but cancer did not hurt them!

Cancer did not destroy our household! It certainly shook things up, and made us hold onto everything that actually matters. We held onto each other, our friends, our church, and our faith! It is now clear to our family what we are most thankful for.

"Train up a child in the way he should go;

even when he is old he will not depart from it." Proverbs 22:6

I have a deeper, more personal understanding of the Bible and can better relate to more of the profound stories and miracles it holds. I learned that the same God, whom King David sang to, is the same wonderful God that I sing to. History and time have passed, but the Lord is forever. His mercies endure forever.

I learned to write down the good stuff. I learned to trust God to use this challenging time to mold me and I hoped to be used for His glory, as well as to benefit others. He convicted me to write these things down. I'm so thankful I did. Looking back at the good things, there were quite a lot of them. Pages and Pages! My journal is an Ebenezer to see how God put people in my life when I needed them for specific times or events and how He lovingly provided for me along the way.

Praise the Lord! Oh give thanks to the Lord, for he is good,

for his steadfast love endures forever! Psalm 106:1

I learned to choose to set my eyes on the Lord and bury my burdens within His Holy Word rather than torment and worry all the time. I can allow His peace to comfort and soothe me. I trust Him and know that whatever comes He will never leave me alone. My relationship and love for the Lord has deepened.

I pray more often and pray for others in a more-committed way. I learned the importance of prayer warriors and how impacting they are. Prayer has been important to me, but having so many others pray for me in this way was new and indescribable. Humbling, touching, comforting, reassuring. I was able to rest better knowing others would be lifting me up, I could relax during tests and know God was with me as people I loved were praying. In dark or frightening moments, peace would come and I'd often find out that someone had felt the need to pray at that moment. Amazing! Knowing what it feels like to be the recipient of prayer support fuels my desire to do the same for others. I believe in the power of prayer and learned to take it more seriously.

"Therefore, confess your sins to one another and pray for one another,

that you may be healed. The prayer of a righteous person

has great power as it is working." James 5:16

I learned to hold tightly to His promises because He never breaks them! I learned to dig into His Word and seek out His promises, plans for His children, and His desires for my life. I learned to study His Word so that I can show my love and devotion to Him through obedience and worship.

I learned to focus on my hope in Christ and the joy and peace His sacrifice brings to my life. I learned to remind myself of what true joy in Him means and to not put so much emphasis on momentary happiness or fleeting emotions. I learned to be still and truly reflect on what the Lord has done, and surrender myself in worship and praise.

I discovered that I have something in common with Apostle Paul. We both have an advantage compared to many; our faith! I felt sad for people who looked unhappy, depressed, or fearful and knew that could have easily been me, if it hadn't been for faith. Knowing that this world is not only the seen or the now, gave me a purpose and joy that cannot be taken away by illness or anything else. I sometimes felt like I was cheating or had the upper hand in learning that cancer is better with faith. My guilt would subside when I'd remember that my "advantage" is available to all.

"For all who are led by the Spirit of God are sons of God. For you did not

receive the spirit of slavery to fall back into fear, but you have received the

Spirit of adoption as sons, by whom we cry, "Abba! Father!" The Spirit

himself bears witness with our spirit that we are children of God, and if

children, then heirs—heirs of God and fellow heirs with Christ, provided

we suffer with him in order that we may also be glorified with him."

Romans 8: 14-17

I learned that illness is hard. Having thought I understood this already, but I now know more about the struggles illness can cause. The physical pain, medical intervention, side effects, scars, appointments, finances, lack of control, mental distress and discouragement... the list continues. It is really hard! But I've become more compassionate towards the physically sick, mentally ill, disabled, and elderly. I realize that none of them want to be restricted by their physical limitations and I can better-relate and have shared something in common with them. I can lend them a listening ear, a smile, or a word of encouragement. Having been the recipient and knowing the value and comfort a bit of compassion can bring.

I learned what a 'good day' is and to appreciate every one of them. Being in hyperbaric treatments really drove this lesson home. Many people are in chronic pain, chronic illness and never get a break! I have a better appreciation knowing that if I am not being poked, prodded, lying in a hospital bed, or have a full belly and a place of safety. That I am having a good day! There are many who would love to trade places with me, so I've learned to be more grateful and appreciate my many good days.

I learned to keep a more present mind-set, and live in the day. I don't worry as much about next year's calendar or what life might bring, because this year taught me everything can change in a day. I am grateful for every day and they all feel like a bonus. I have been given the gift of life and don't want to misuse or squander it.

My appreciation for God's creation of life has deepened. Mine, my families, the birds, the flowers - they are here today and may be gone tomorrow, so I want to gaze at them, study them, and enjoy them!

Life can change so quickly and I am overjoyed to be here with my family. *Now* is the time! I try not to procrastinate on the good, meaningful stuff. I am reminded to actively listen to my children when they speak, pay attention to their giggles, and enjoy our daily life. Celebrate every success, encourage, and build each other up! I've learned to not waste any time on negativity or foolishness. Life does not have a pause or rewind button, so now I make an effort to use my time more wisely!

"For everything there is a season, and a time for every matter under heaven"

Ecclesiastes 3:1

My love and appreciation for music has grown. I listen more closely to song lyrics and I ponder the words like poetry. Music often moves me to tears. I sing louder, unashamedly. I found that singing praise is its own form of daily devotion, and that it sometimes leads me straight to scripture.

"Make a joyful noise to the LORD, all the earth; break forth into joyous song and sing praises! Sing praises to the LORD with the lyre, with the lyre and the sound of melody! With trumpets and the sound of the horn make a joyful noise before the King, the LORD!" Psalm 98:4-6

I've found more reasons to laugh. I value quality time with friends. I learned more about friendship and what it means to lift each other's burdens. I know more about the powerful expression of love that a prayer offered can show. That a text message sent with care can cast out loneliness, or a card mailed can lift one's spirit over and over, and that encouraging words are healing. I've learned the value of a good listener and that a comforting hug cannot be measured. That tears really never run dry, but prayers and a shoulder to cry on help them stop faster! I've seen the love that is poured into a hot meal or freshly-prepped vegetables. I learned to express my care for others more easily and to show appreciation at every possible opportunity.

I learned that the two short words "thank you" are powerful and meaningful. It seems like a small gesture, but every person who has a job to do or who helps needs to be thanked. It brightens everyone's day to be appreciated. I learned that gratitude multiplies gratitude and to "throw around kindness like confetti!". A little kindness speaks volumes! It intrigued me to see how strangers respond and quickly open up when offered even the smallest kindness.

"But God demonstrates his own love for us in this:

While we were still sinners, Christ died for us." Romans 5:8

Most of all, more than ever before, I now know that I am truly loved and valuable! I am loved more than I thought possible. This might be the best lesson I learned from cancer. This is a lesson I wish everyone could experience without the trial. When I got this diagnosis, it very quickly became obvious to me that I am loved and lots more people care about me than I'd ever noticed. The Lord showed me His love in these lessons, His presence and His peace.

Cancer changed me and every day something reminds me of what my family learned last year. Some days the memories bring tears and some days they bring smiles. I hope that I never forget what happened because I learned more in that year than I ever thought possible. Becoming a survivor is an honor. It's an honor that not every cancer patient is able to experience, but for this opportunity and these lessons I am forever grateful!

Praise to God for a Living Hope

"Praise be to the God and Father of our Lord Jesus Christ! In his great mercy he has given us new birth into a living hope through the resurrection of Jesus Christ from the dead, and into an inheritance that can never perish, spoil or fade. This inheritance is kept in heaven for you, who through faith are shielded by God's power until the coming of the salvation that is ready to be revealed in the last time. In all this you greatly rejoice, though now for a little while you may have had to suffer grief in all kinds of trials. These have come so that the proven genuineness of your faith—of greater worth than gold, which perishes even though refined by fire—may result in praise, glory and honor when Jesus Christ is revealed. Though you have not seen him, you love him; and even though you do not see him now, you believe in him and are filled with an inexpressible and glorious joy, for you are receiving the end result of your faith, the salvation of your souls."

1 Peter 1: 3-9

LAURA PENTSA

LAURA PENTSA

ABOUT THE AUTHOR

Laura Pentsa and her husband, Dave, have three full spirited, fun loving children. They live in Phoenix, AZ where her husband is pastor at a local Christian church. Cancer is only a small part of their lives together, but it has left many valuable imprints on their family. Laura has since joined the non-profit organization, "Don't Be a Chump! Check For a Lump" their mission is to educate women on breast health awareness and prevention of breast cancer to help save lives! They also offer direct assistance to breast cancer patients in Arizona with free wigs. For more information visit checkforalump.org

LAURA PENTSA

English Standard Version. Bible Gateway. Web. 5 July 2017.